The Handbook of Office Urological Procedures

Hashim Hashim, Paul Abrams, and
Roger Dmochowski (Eds.)

The Handbook of Office Urological Procedures

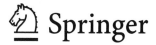 Springer

Hashim Hashim, MBBS, MRCS
Urology Specialist Registrar
Bristol Urological Institute
Southmead Hospital
Bristol
UK

Paul Abrams, MD, FRCS
Professor of Urology
Bristol Urological Institute
Southmead Hospital
Bristol
UK

Roger Dmochowski, MD, FACS
Professor of Urology
Vanderbilt University Medical Center
Nashville, TN
USA

British Library Cataloguing in Publication Data

The handbook of office urological procedures
  1. Urology   2. Genitourinary organs – Diseases – Diagnosis
  3. Genitourinary organs – Surgery
  I. Hashim, Hashim   II. Abrams, Paul, 1947–   III. Dmochowski,
  Roger R.
  616.6

ISBN-13: 9781846285233

Library of Congress Control Number: 2007927935

ISBN: 978-1-84628-523-3   e-ISBN: 978-1-84628-706-0

9 8 7 6 5 4 3 2 1

Springer Science+Business Media
springer.com

Foreword

Urology is a branch of surgery dealing with diseases of the urinary tract. Over the past decade, there has been a shift in the practice of urology toward a more "office"-based service. Depending on the type of practice one has, up to 80% of urological surgery can be dealt with on an ambulatory day-case basis, either in the hospital or in the office, with emphasis on diagnostic and minor or intermediate surgical procedures. Major urological surgery is becoming concentrated in only relatively few centers in every country.

This handbook of office urological procedures deals in an orderly fashion with the common core urological procedures that every urologist needs to be competent at doing, as they form the "bread-and-butter" of urological practice.

The book is divided into 31 chapters with illustrations to illustrate the practical procedures encountered in daily urological practice. These procedures are often "submerged" in the large textbooks by the specialized discussions on topics like prostate cancer. However, being a pocket-sized book, the handbook can be carried around easily by trainees.

I congratulate the authors on their hard work in producing a book which will help to educate physicians and improve patient care.

Alan J. Wein, MD, PhD (Hon)
University of Pennsylvania Health System
Philadelphia, PA, USA

Preface

Time constraints on the undergraduate curriculum and changes in patients' attitudes have resulted in medical students and doctors-in-training receiving reduced formal teaching and acquiring fewer practical skills than their predecessors. This can mean that many doctors have very limited experience of even the common diagnostic tests and surgical procedures that they are likely to encounter in their day-to-day practice as trainees. For the doctor expected to perform urological procedures with which he or she has had limited experience, this book will be an invaluable source of information and advice.

The procedures in this book are often embedded in larger operative textbooks that are difficult to carry around. These larger textbooks also cover all aspects of urological surgery, some of which, such as radical prostatectomy, are useful to know about, but are usually performed in specialist centers and not on a regular basis by general "core/office" urologists.

This book provides a practical and comprehensive summary of the most common "office" urological procedures in a form that is concise, relevant, readily available, and easily carried around. The chapters are organized in an orderly fashion, starting with the equipment used by urologists. This is followed by operative and investigative procedures of the genitalia and ends with procedures on the upper urinary tract.

The book was written with urological trainees in mind but we hope it would also be useful for medical students, general surgical trainees, and general practitioners with a special interest in urology as well as practicing urologists.

Hashim Hashim
Bristol, UK
2008

Acknowledgments

We are grateful for all those who helped us to produce this book, especially the medical equipment companies including Laborie, Olympus, Karl-Storz, Cook, Bard, and Coloplast who provided illustrations for the book. We would also like to thank Alice Chen for drawing the illustrations.

Hashim Hashim
Paul Abrams
Roger Dmochowski

Contents

Contributors

Paul Abrams, MD, FRCS
Professor of Urology
Bristol Urological Institute
Southmead Hospital
Bristol, UK

Roger Dmochowski, MD, FACS
Professor of Urology
Vanderbilt University Medical Center
Nashville, TN
USA

Hashim Hashim MBBS, MRCS
Urology Specialist Registrar
Bristol Urological Institute
Southmead Hospital
Bristol, UK

Christopher Wolter MD
Instructor in Urology
Vanderbilt University Medical Center
Nashville, TN
USA

1. Sutures and Scalpels

Hashim Hashim

Sutures

Sutures form an integral part of any surgeon's tools, and therefore the surgeon needs to be familiar with the physical characteristics and properties of sutures. The choice of suture depends on the anatomical site, the surgeon's preference, and the required suture characteristics, which include:

1. Degradation
2. Structure
3. Material type
4. Color
5. Size
6. Coating
7. Mounting

Degradation

Sutures can be either absorbable or non-absorbable. Absorbable sutures are degraded and broken down by hydrolysis, if synthetic, or proteolysis, if natural, after a period of time that can range from a few days to months and years. Hydrolysis causes less tissue reaction. Absorbable sutures provide only temporary wound support until the wound heals. Non-absorbable sutures are not metabolized by the body, do not dissolve, and are permanent. They cause a tissue reaction in which fibroblasts encapsulate the suture.

Structure

Suture structure can be monofilament or multi-filament. Monofilament sutures are made of single strands. They tend to be smooth and therefore slide well in tissues. But if handled inappropriately (e.g., crushed), they can fracture, weaken, and lead to premature suture failure.

Multi-filament sutures are composed of multiple filaments and may be twisted or braided. They are easier to handle than monofilaments and therefore easier to tie and knot because they have a higher coefficient of friction. They have a greater surface area and increased capillarity, therefore having a greater tendency to absorb fluid and harbor bacteria.

Material Type

Different materials have been used to make sutures. They can be natural or synthetic. Synthetic sutures include: polyglycolic acid, polyglactin, polydioxone, polyglyconate, polyamide, polyester, and polypropylene. Natural sutures include: stainless steel, silk, catgut, and linen. Please note that in Europe and Japan, gut sutures have been banned because of concerns over bovine spongiform encephalopathy (BSE), although the herds from which gut is harvested are certified BSE-free.

Color

Sutures can be dyed or undyed. Undyed sutures do not stain and are therefore used mainly for the skin layer.

Size

The gauge of sutures is expressed in numbers using the United States Pharmacopeia (USP) gauge or metric gauge. The USP gauge refers to the diameter of the suture strand and is denoted by zeroes. The more zeroes the smaller the diameter and the lower the tensile strength (e.g., 4/0 [4-0 or 0000] is smaller than 2/0 [2-0 or 00]). Table 1 shows how USP compares to the metric system.

Coating

Sutures can be coated or uncoated. Coating materials include: wax, silicone, polyvinyl solution, magnesium stearate, vinyl acetate, polybutilate, or glyconate.

Table 1.1. USP Versus the Metric Diameter of Sutures.

USP Designation	Collagen metric diameter (mm)	Synthetic absorbable metric diameter (mm)	Non-absorbable metric diameter (mm)
11-0			0.01
10-0	0.02	0.02	0.02
9-0	0.03	0.03	0.03
8-0	0.05	0.04	0.04
7-0	0.07	0.05	0.05
6-0	0.1	0.07	0.07
5-0	0.15	0.1	0.1
4-0	0.2	0.15	0.15
3-0	0.3	0.2	0.2
2-0	0.35	0.3	0.3
0	0.4	0.35	0.35
1	0.5	0.4	0.4
2	0.6	0.5	0.5
3	0.7	0.6	0.6
4	0.8	0.6	0.6
5		0.7	0.7
6			0.8
7			

Mounting

Sutures may be mounted on needles or unmounted. Mounted sutures are used to close wounds, whereas unmounted sutures are mainly used to tie blood vessels.

Other Physical Characteristics of Sutures

1. Tensile strength – Measure of a material or tissue's ability to resist deformation and breakage. Weight necessary to break a suture divided

Table 1.2. Examples of Sutures.

	Absorbable	Non-absorbable
Natural monofilament		Stainless steel
Natural multi-filament	Catgut – plain or chromic	Silk Linen
Synthetic monofilament	Polydioxanone (PDS)	Polyamide (Nylon)
	Polyglyconate (Maxon)	Polypropylene (Prolene)
Synthetic multi-filament	Polyglactin (Vicryl)	Polyester (Dacron)
	Polyglycolic acid (Dexon)	

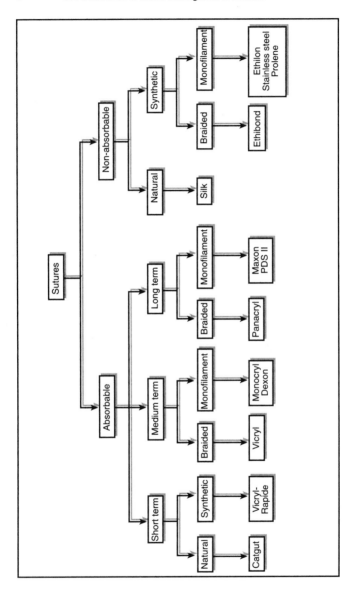

Figure 1.1. Which Suture Would You Choose?

by the sutures cross-sectional area (mm^2). A knotted suture has one-third the strength of an unknotted suture. The greater the number of throws in a knot, the less the tensile strength. Polyester and polypropylene have the best tensile strength, whereas silk has the weakest.

2. Capillarity – Ability of a suture to absorb fluid.
3. Elasticity – Ability of a suture to regain its original form and length after deformation.
4. Knot strength – Force necessary to cause a knot to slip either partially or fully. It is dependent on the coefficient of static friction and plasticity.
5. Memory – Inherent capability of suture to return to or maintain its original gross shape (related to elasticity, plasticity, and diameter).
6. Plasticity – Ability of a suture to retain its new form after release of the deforming force.
7. Pliability – Ability to adjust knot tension and to secure knots (i.e., handling ability).
8. Memory – Ability of a suture to return to its original shape after deformation.

Needles

Needles come in a variety of types, shapes, lengths, and diameters, with a suture attached to it through a drilled hole. The size of the needle depends on the size of the suture. The choice of needle depends on several factors, including the requirements of the specific procedure, the nature of the tissue to be sutured, the accessibility of the operative area, and the preferred techniques of the individual surgeon.

Every needle can be described by its anatomy.

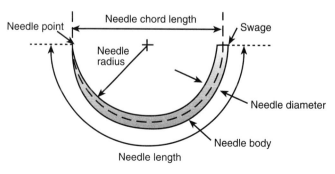

Figure 1.2.

1. **Needle point**
   The needle point is the portion of the needle that extends from the tip to the maximum cross-section of the body. Three main types of points exist:
   A. Cutting
   Required wherever fibrous or dense tissue needs to be sutured.
   - Conventional cutting needle
     - Triangular cross-section
     - Apex of triangle is on the on the inner, concave curvature (surface-seeking)
     - Upward-pointing triangle

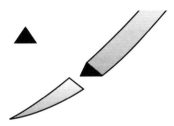

Figure 1.3.

   - Reverse cutting needle
     - Triangular cross-section
     - Apex cutting edge on the outer convex curvature of the needle (depth-seeking)
     - Downward-pointing triangle

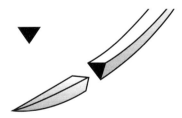

Figure 1.4.

   - Trocar-point needle
     - Strong cutting head
     - Round body

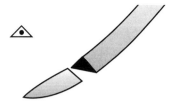

Figure 1.5.

B. Round-bodied
Designed to separate tissue fibers rather than cut them (e.g., for soft tissue or in situations where easy splitting of tissue fibers is possible). They are conical with a circular cross-section.
- Taper-point needle
  - Forceps flats are formed in an area half way between the point and attachment
  - A sharp tip at the point flattens to an oval/rectangular shape
  - Sharpness is determined by taper ratio and tip angle. The needle is sharper if it has a higher taper ratio and lower tip angle.

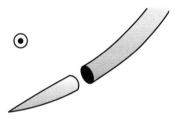

Figure 1.6.

- Blunt-point needle
  - Minimize the risk of needle stick injury
  - Sharp enough to penetrate fascia and muscle but not skin
  - Suturing friable tissue such as the liver

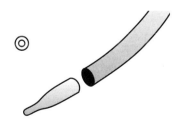

Figure 1.7.

C. Spatula needle
  • Side-cutting
    • Flat on the top and bottom surfaces to reduce tissue injury
    • Mainly for ophthalmic procedures

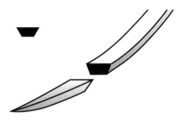

Figure 1.8.

2. **Body**
   The majority of the needle length is body. The body is what interacts with the needle holder. Interaction affected by needle diameter and radius, body geometry, and stainless steel alloy. The body can be:
   • Flatted: allows for stability in the needle holder.
   • Ribbed: allows larger needles to provide a secure grip.
   • Square: allows for increased needle strength.
3. **Swage**
   A hole is drilled into the end of the wire and the material is attached into this hole in a continuous fashion.
   • Channel swage: Suture introduced into a channel in the needle with the diameter of the channel swage greater than the diameter of the needle body.
   • Drill swage: The diameter of the drill swage is less than the diameter of the needle body.
   • Nonswaged: Suture is passed through an eye instead of a swage.
4. **Needle coating**
   The needle may be coated with silicone to permit easier tissue passage with less friction.
5. **Needle measurements**
   • Chord length: Linear distance from the point of the curved needle to the swage (bite width).
   • Needle length: Distance measured along the needle from the point to the swage. It is the measurement supplied on suture packages.
   • Radius: Distance from the body of the needle to the center of the circle along which the needle curves (bite depth).
   • Diameter: The gauge or thickness of the needle wire is considered the diameter.
6. **Needle body shape**
   There are many different needle shapes. Choice of needle shape is frequently governed by the accessibility of the tissue to be sutured, and normally the more confined the operative site the greater the curvature required.

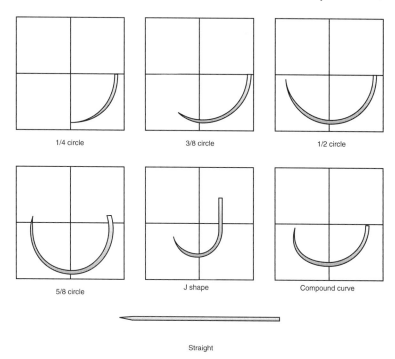

1/4 circle   3/8 circle   1/2 circle

5/8 circle   J shape   Compound curve

Straight

Figure 1.9.

- Straight: Used for easily accessible tissue that can be manipulated directly by hand (e.g., subcuticular skin).
- Curved: Has a predictable path through tissue and requires less space for maneuvering than a straight needle.
- Compound curved: Has 80° curvature at the tip and 45° curvature throughout the remainder of the body. Used mainly in microvascular and ophthalmic surgery.

Scalpels and Holders

The most common blades used in urology are numbers 10, 11, and 15.

1. No. 10 scalpels have a large curved edge and are mainly used for large incisions, such as when access is required to the abdomen.
2. No. 11 scalpels have a pointed edge and are used for stab incisions, such as when incising and draining an abscess.

3. No. 15 scalpels have a small curved cutting edge and are used for performing scrotal surgery.
4. All the above blades can be placed on a No. 3 scalpel holder.

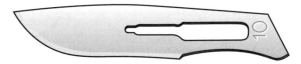

Figure 1.10. No. 10 blade.

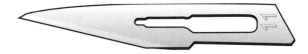

Figure 1.11. No. 11 blade.

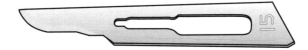

Figure 1.12. No. 15 blade.

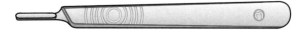

Figure 1.13. No. 3 scalpel holder.

References

1. Taylor B, Bayat A. Basic plastic surgery techniques and principles: choosing the right suture material. Student BMJ 2003;11:140–141.
2. Bennett RG. Selection of wound closure materials. J Am Acad Dermatol 1988;18(4 Pt 1):619–637.
3. http://www.ethiconproducts.co.uk.

2. Electrosurgical Diathermy

Hashim Hashim

Principles of Diathermy

- High frequency ALTERNATING current
- Safe current up to 500 mA
- Frequency of 400 kHz to 10 MHz
- Produced by a generator/machine
- Local temperatures up to 1000°C
- No stimulation to neuromuscular tissue

Types of Diathermy

1. **Monopolar**
   - High-power unit (400 W)
   - High-frequency current
   - Active electrode held by surgeon (HIGH current density)
     - Point forceps
     - Spatula
     - Diathermy scissors
   - Patient plate (indifferent/dispersive/neutral/passive/return) electrode (LOW current density)
     - Good contact (at least 70 cm^2 for minimal heating)
     - Dry surface, avoid kinking
     - Shaved skin (thigh or back)
     - Avoid bony prominences and scar tissue (poor blood supply $\Rightarrow$ poor heat distribution)
     - Avoid areas where there are metal prostheses (e.g., total hip replacement)
     - Alarm system if there is fault
   - May earth away from the plate
   - May channel the current, resulting in a pedicle effect: Electric current passing from target organ to connected adjoining tissue via small delicate structures causing heating of the structure to the extent that tissue damage can occur, resulting in partial or total occlusion of the vessel lumen.
   - May cause explosions in or out of the patient

- Causes little charring
- Least effective on fat
- Active electrode can either be hand- or foot-activated
- Electrode tips
  - Loops to cut and fulgurate
  - Ball electrodes for desiccation (contact coagulation) and fulguration (non-contact coagulation)
  - Needles and blades to cut and coagulate

2. **Bipolar**
   - Low-power unit (50 W)
   - Frequency between 250 kHz and 1 MHz
   - Current passes between limbs of insulated forceps only, with reduced damage to surrounding tissue
   - No patient plate electrode
   - Safer than monopolar because current does not pass through the body of the patient and only through the tissue grasped between the tips of the forceps
   - Less effective in cutting and needs special design to cut and coagulate
   - Useful on narrow pedicles (i.e., penis, digits)
   - Tends to char
   - Slower than monopolar because each vessel has to be grasped and coagulated separately
   - Greater coagulation efficiency because pressure exerted on a blood vessel by forceps increases heat dissipation and desiccation
   - Can be hand- or foot-activated

Generators (Figure 2.1)

1. **Earth-referenced**
   - Older type
   - Wide/High frequency range (>1 MHz)
   - Earth leakage unavoidable
   - Capacitor earthing
   - Still works if no patient plate electrode: current division occurs by finding an alternate pathway
   - Zero potential at patient plate electrode
2. **Isolated/floating**
   - Modern, smaller
   - Tight frequency range (400–600 kHz)
   - Reduced earth leakage
   - Uses transistors
   - Not earthed
   - Does NOT work without patient plate electrode
   - No patient plate electrode ⇒ no current

Mode Settings

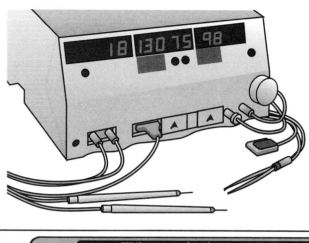

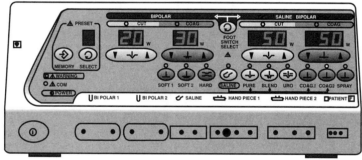

Figure 2.1. Electrosurgery Unit.

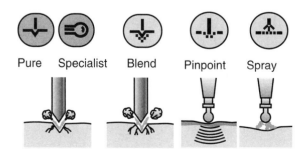

Figure 2.2. Diagram of Different Mode Settings.

1. Cutting

- Pure or specialist
- Continuous output
- Unmodulated sine wave
- Low voltages can be used
- Forms small continuous arc between the electrode and the tissue
- Causes rapid cell destruction followed by the complete explosion of the cell with water vaporization
- Causes tissue disruption
- Some vessel coagulation is achieved if electrode is placed directly on tissue (desiccation)
- Specialist cut mode is for operations in wet fields (fluid), which have increased levels of conductivity because of the wet environment. Delivers more power into higher resistances
- 125–250 W

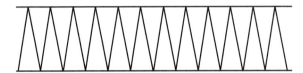

Scheme 2.1.

2. Blend

- Only works in cutting mode
- Provides coagulation at the same time as cutting
- Not a continuous waveform
- Higher voltage used than pure cut
- Superimposed burst of high frequency
- Increases hemostasis

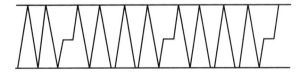

Scheme 2.2.

3. Coagulation

- Pulsed output, short intervals: current is "off" for longer periods than it is "on"
- Much higher voltages required
- Modulated sine wave

- Minimum tissue disruption
- Vessel coagulation
- Water vaporization
- Desiccation (pinpoint or contact coagulation): creates rapid localized heat at the end of the blood vessel, causing contraction with eventual occlusion of the lumen.
- Fulgaration (spray coagulation)
  - Electrode is not in contact with tissue (2–4 mm away)
  - Creates an air gap across which the current must jump
  - More widespread coagulation than other coagulation modes
  - Should not be used in laparoscopic or endoscopic surgery
  - Higher voltages could break down the insulation of the instruments used
- 40–75 W

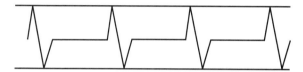

Scheme 2.3.

General Safety Principles

- Patient should not be touching earthed metal
- Avoid pooling of inflammable agents
- Use lowest practicable power setting
- Make sure the active electrode in contact with target tissue is in view
- Keep the plate away from metallic implants

Reference

1. Eschmann Equipment Home. http://www.eschmann.co.uk. Date accessed: May 25, 2007.

3. Urinary Catheters

Hashim Hashim

Indications

Urinary catheters are used to drain urine from the bladder. The main indications are:

A. **Diagnostic**
  - Measure post-void residual in the absence of ultrasound scanning
  - Urine sample for evaluation by culture and microscopy in patients who are unable to void
  - Measure urine output in critically ill patients

B. **Investigational**
  - Filling the bladder prior to ultrasound investigation of the abdomen
  - Urodynamics
  - Cystograms

C. **Therapeutic**
  - During labor when epidural anaesthesia is used
  - Urinary retention (e.g., secondary to bladder outlet obstruction)
  - Intractable urinary incontinence
  - Major surgery (e.g., hip surgery, abdominal and pelvic surgery)
  - Instillation of chemotherapeutic agents (e.g., mitomycin C and bacillus Calmette-Guérin [BCG])
  - Patients who are not fit for or do not want medical or surgical treatment for their bladder conditions

Methods of Bladder Catheterization

Four methods of draining or collecting urine from the bladder exist. Their use depends on patient's condition, availability of catheters, as well as local expertise and support.

1. Condom catheters: A condom is attached to the catheter and a drainage bag so that men can void through the penis into the condom and the urine is collected in the drainage bag.
2. Clean intermittent self-catheterization (CISC): Uses lubricated sterile catheters that are inserted by the patient though the urethra on an as

required basis to drain urine. They need manual dexterity to be inserted.

3. Intra-urethral catheterization: These are self-retaining catheters used to continuously drain urine from the bladder and inserted via the urethra.

4. Suprapubic catheterization: A catheter is inserted through the skin in the lower anterior abdominal wall and into the bladder (*see* Chapter 25).

Classification of Urinary Catheters

Intra-urethral and suprapubic catheters can be classified according to their size, material, type of tip, position of holes, number of lumens, as well as the number and volume of inflatable balloons. There are also catheters without balloons.

A. **Size**

Many catheter sizes are available. The choice depends on the patient and the indication of use. Size is measured in:
- Charrière (Ch) units: catheter's *diameter* in millimeters (1 Ch = 0.33 mm diameter
- French (Fr) units: catheter's *circumference* in millimeters (12 Fr = 12-mm circumference)

The length of catheters can be:
- Pediatric: 30 cm
- Female: 26 cm (20–26 cm)
- Standard: 43 cm (41–54 cm)
- You should only use standard catheters for men.

B. **Material**
- Latex (rubber)
  - Soft and flexible
  - All rubber uncoated: short-term use up to 4 weeks
    - Does not have a smooth surface, causing high surface friction
  - Polytetrafluoroethylene (PTFE)-coated
    - Inert
    - Provides a smooth outer surface
    - Can remain *in situ* for up to 4 weeks
  - Silicone elastomer-coated
    - Less prone to encrustation
    - Compatible with the urethral mucosa
    - Can remain *in situ* for up to 12 weeks
  - Hydrogel-coated
    - Absorb fluid, thus form a hydrophilic slippery "cushion" between urethra and catheter surface reducing trauma
    - Resists encrustation and bacterial colonisation
    - Can remain *in situ* for up to 12 weeks

- Silver-alloy coated: can reduce infections in the short-term
- Silicone
  - 100% latex free: used in those with latex allergy
  - Thin-walled
  - Have wider drainage lumens
  - Compatible with the urethral mucosa
  - Lack flexibility
  - High surface friction
  - Can remain *in situ* for up to 12 weeks
  - Can be hydrogel coated
- Plastic or polyvinylchloride (PVC)
  - Relatively cheap
  - Develop cracks and quickly encrust
  - Short-term use (e.g., CISC)
  - Rigid at temperatures lower than body temperature and therefore can cause discomfort
  - Thin-walled with the widest lumens
- C. **Tip and Holes (Figure 3.1)**
  - Straight: no bends at the tip
    - Ordinary straight: holes on the side
    - Couvelaire (whistle-tip): straight with openings lateral and distal to the balloon, providing a large drainage area to drain debris and blood clots
    - Council tip: have a small hole at the tip, which allows them to be passed over a wire

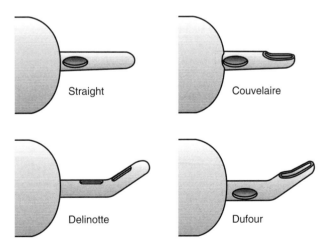

Figure 3.1. Catheter Tips and Holes.

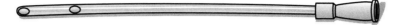

Figure 3.2. Single-Lumen Catheters.

- Coude: Bent/curved tip (approximately 45°) to allow passage through prostate
  - Delinotte (Mercier): a bent straight-tip
  - Dufour: a bent couvelaire
- **D. Lumens**
  - One lumen
    - Nelaton catheters (Figure 3.2): a simple straight tube with (a) hole(s) at the end. These are mainly used for CISC. These catheters do not normally have an inflatable balloon.
    - Malécot or DePezzer catheters (Figure 3.3): These have a triangular-/mushroom-looking tip designed for suprapubic catheterization or to drain urine from the renal pelvis. They are without a balloon, and therefore will stay in position because the tip will fold out once the stick inside the lumen of the catheter is retracted.
  - Two lumens (Figures 3.4)

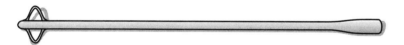

Figure 3.3. Malecot Catheter.

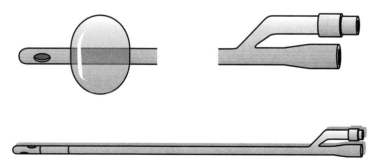

Figure 3.4. Two-Way Foley Catheter with Balloon Inflated and Deflated.

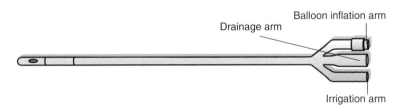

Figure 3.5. Three-Way Catheter.

- Foley catheters: Two-way catheters with a tube and a balloon at the end to keep them from falling out of the bladder.
- Three lumens (Figure 3.5)
  - Hemostatic catheters: Three-way catheters are generally thicker than the previous two catheters with an extra small separate channel. This allows fluid/irrigant to pass to the tip of the catheter and into the bladder to flush it and wash away blood and small clots through the primary arm that drains into a collection device. The inflation arm has a small plastic valve that allows for the introduction or removal of sterile water through a very small channel to inflate or deflate the retaining balloon.
- Four lumens (Figure 3.6)

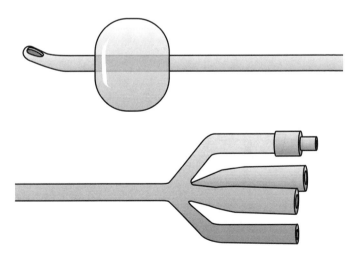

Figure 3.6. Four-Way Catheter.

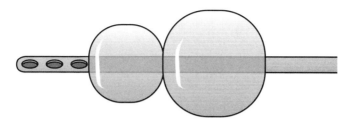

Figure 3.7. Two-Balloon Catheter.

- Three of the four lumens act as drainage conduit, inflation and deflation valve, or continuous irrigation port while the fourth lumen provides irrigation or aspiration of the operative site (e.g., following a transurethral resection of the prostate).
E. **Number and Volume of Balloons**
  - The maximum volume the balloon can accommodate is normally printed on the side of one of the arms. This can range from 5–40 mL.
  - Most catheters have one balloon; however, there are some catheters that have two balloons (Figure 3.7). They are normally used after prostatectomy, and the second balloon sits in the prostatic capsule/fossa to help with tamponade of bleeding vessels. The bladder balloon is generally inflated first and the catheter pulled to the bladder neck and then the prostatic balloon is inflated.

Complications of Urinary Catheters

- Discomfort
- Bladder spasms
- Catheter-associated urinary tract infections
- Trauma resulting in urethral strictures, false passages, and hematuria
- Bowel injury and perforation of the bladder
- Paraphimosis
- Urine leakage around the catheter
- Calculi formation

- Fragmentation and fracture of the catheter
- Bladder cancer in long-term use of catheters (rare)

Reference

1. Ramakrishnan K, Mold JW. Urinary catheters: a review. Internet J Fam Pract 2005;Vol 3;2.

4. Urological Endoscopic Equipment

Hashim Hashim

This chapter will show pictures of common equipment that are used by a urologist and is not covered in other chapters.

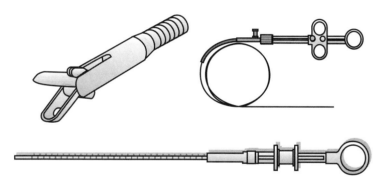

Figure 4.1. Flexible Biopsy Forceps Used to Take Biopsies During Flexible Cystoscopy.

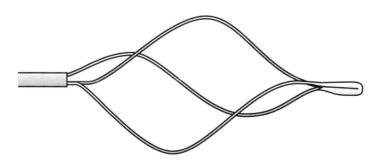

Figure 4.2. Basket Used to Remove Stones in the Ureter.

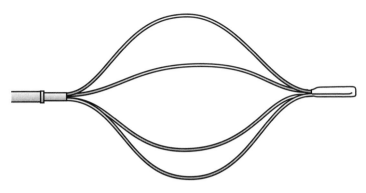

Figure 4.2. (*Continued*)

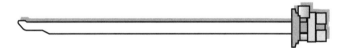

Figure 4.3. Cystoscope Sheath With Beak.

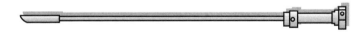

Figure 4.4. Obturator Used to Aid Insertion of the Sheath.

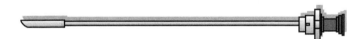

Figure 4.5. Optical Obturator Uses a Camera to Aid Insertion of Sheath into the Bladder.

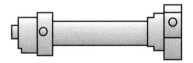

Figure 4.6. Bridge.

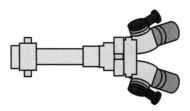

Figure 4.7. Two-Way Bridge.

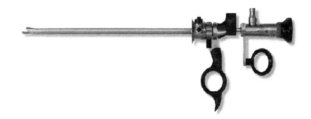

Figure 4.8. Rigid Biopsy Forceps.

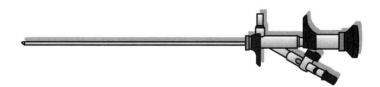

Figure 4.9. Straight Ocular Cystosocpe.

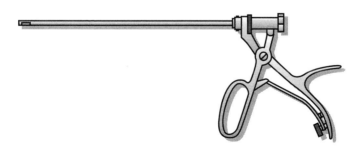

Figure 4.10. Optical Stone Punch Used to Crush Stones in the Bladder Under Vision.

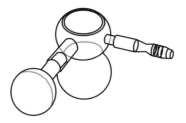

Figure 4.11. Ellick Evacuator Used to Evacuate Clots, Debris, and Prostate or Bladder Chips Following Resection.

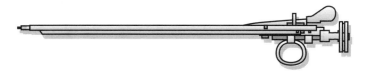

Figure 4.12. Otis Urethrotome.

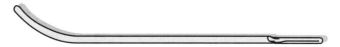

Figure 4.13. Curved Metal Sounds Used to Dilate the Urethra in Men.

Replacement of original brief of a penile clamp

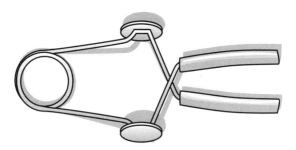

Figure 4.14. Strauss Penile Clamp Used to Stop Male Leakage.

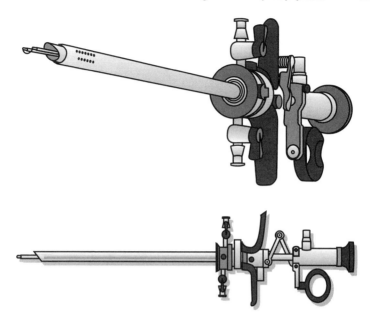

Figure 4.15. Continuous Irrigation Resectoscope Used for Transurethral Resection of Prostate or Bladder Tumor (TURP/TURBT).

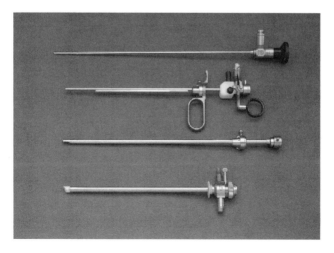

Figure 4.16. Different Parts of a Resectoscope.

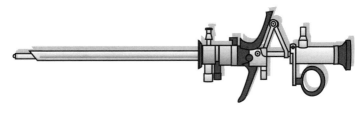

Figure 4.17. Intermittent Irrigation Resectoscope.

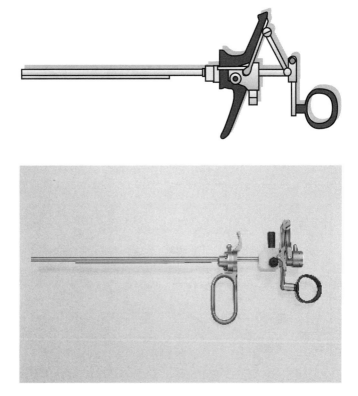

Figure 4.18. Resectoscope Working Element.

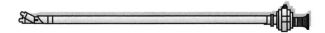

Figure 4.19. Resectoscope Inner Sheath With Deflector Obturator Tip.

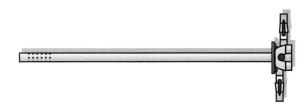

Figure 4.20. Outer Sheath.

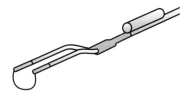

Figure 4.21. Resection Loop Electrode Used for TURP/TURBT.

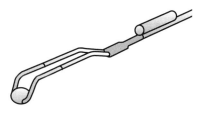

Figure 4.22. Roller Electrode Used to Coagulate Vessels Following TURP/TURBT.

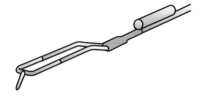

Figure 4.23. Needle Electrode Used for Bladder Neck Incision.

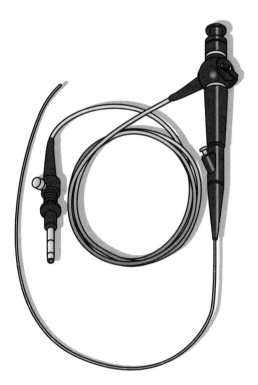

Figure 4.24. Flexible Ureteroscope.

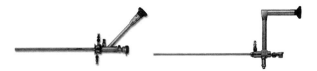

Figure 4.25. Nephroscope.

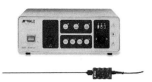

Figure 4.26. Electrohydraulic (EHL) and Electrokinetic (EKL) Lithotriptor.

5. Local Anesthesia and Nerve Blocks

Hashim Hashim

Indications

Many inguino-scrotal procedures in urology can be performed under local anesthesia. Sometimes local anesthetics are used to supplement post-operative pain relief in patients who had general anesthesia. The common nerve blocks are an inguinal block for hernia repairs and inguinal orchidectomies, a cord block for vasectomies, and a penile block for circumcision and frenuloplasty. The testis and scrotum are innervated by the ilioinguinal, genitofemoral, pudendal, and posterior scrotal nerves. L1-S3 provide the autonomic nerve supply; T10-L4 provide the sympathetic nervous system; and S1-S3 provide the parasympathetic nerve supply. The penis is supplied by the dorsal nerve and the posterior scrotal branches of the pudendal nerve, as well as the ilioinguinal, genitofemoral, and posterior cutaneous nerve of the thigh.

Types of Local Anesthetics

The two main local anesthetics used are lidocaine (to provide rapid anesthesia) or bupivicaine (to provide prolonged anesthesia) (Table 5.1). Epinephrine can be added to these anesthetic agents to decrease the rate of absorption and toxicity and to extend duration of action; however, its use should be avoided in the extremities as it may cause ischemia.

Drug concentration is expressed on a percentage which is measured in grams per 100 mL e.g. 0.5% of bupivicaine = 0.5 g/100mL = 500 mg/100mL = 5 mg/mL. Relationship between concentration, volume, and dose: Concentration (%) × Volume (mL) × 10 = Dose (mg)

The maximum safe dose of epinephrine is 0.25 mg and is normally denoted as weight (g) per volume of solution (mL). For example:

1 : 80,000 = 1 g in 80,000 mL = 1 mg in 80 mL = 12.5/g/mL
1 : 200,000 = 1 g in 200,000 mL = 1 mg in 200 mL = 5/g/mL
(i.e., 20 mL of 1 : 80,000 or 50 mL of 1 : 200,000)

Inguinal Block

1. Withdraw your local anesthetic into a 20-mL syringe using a 21 G (0.81-mm outer diameter) 1.5-inch needle, then dispose of the needle accordingly.

Table 5.1. Comparison of Lidocaine and Bupivicaine.

	LIDOCAINE	BUPIVICAINE
Dose	3 mg/kg	2 mg/kg
Maximum dose	200 mg	150 mg
Dose with epinephrine	6 mg/kg	2 mg/kg
Maximum dose with epinephrine	500 mg	150 mg
Onset of action	Rapid (~2 mins)	Up to 40 min
Duration of action	60–180 min	2–3 hrs

2. Infiltrate the skin subcutaneously along the intended incision line, if the procedure is being done under local anesthesia, using 25 G (0.51-mm outer diameter) 1-inch needle.
3. Palpate the anterior superior iliac spine and locate the point 2 cm medial to it.
4. Attach and insert a 21 G 2-inch needle perpendicular to and through the skin. In overweight patients a long 120-mm spinal needle can be used instead.
5. Keep on inserting the needle. You will feel the needle "giving way" or feel a "pop." This happens when the needle passes through the aponeurosis of the external oblique.
6. Aspirate for blood. If negative, inject approximately one-quarter of the local anesthetic to block the iliohypogastric nerve.
7. Insert the needle deeper to pass through the internal oblique, aspirate to check that there is no blood, and then inject another quarter of the local anesthetic between the internal oblique and transversus abdominis to block the ilioinguinal nerve.
8. Insert the needle deeper, aspirate to check that there is no blood, and then inject superior to the aponeurosis to block the cutaneous nerve supply from the inferior and subcostal nerves.
9. Now palpate the deep internal inguinal ring (1–1.5 cm above the midpoint of the inguinal ligament).
10. Insert the needle into the inguinal canal and aspirate for blood.
11. If negative, inject approximately 5 mL of local anesthetic to block the genital branch of the genitofemoral nerve.
12. Remove the syringe and needle and insert it approximately 2 cm above and slightly lateral to the pubic tubercle and inject the remaining local anesthetic to block any contralateral nerve innervations.

Spermatic Cord Block

1. Withdraw your local anesthetic into a 20-mL syringe using a 21 G 1.5-inch needle, then dispose of the needle accordingly.
2. Infiltrate the skin subcutaneously along the intended incision line, if the procedure is being done under local anesthesia, using 25 G 1-inch needle.
3. Identify the pubic tubercle.

4. Attach and insert a 21 G 2-inch needle 1 cm below and medial to the pubic tubercle until you reach bone.
5. Withdraw needle slightly and aspirate. If no blood is aspirated, inject about three-quarters of the local anesthetic in different directions in that area.
6. Leave one-quarter of the local anesthetic in the syringe, as you may need to infiltrate the local area as you proceed with the procedure.

OR

1. Withdraw your local anesthetic into a 20-mL syringe using a 21 G 1.5-inch needle, then dispose of the needle accordingly.
2. Infiltrate the skin subcutaneously along the intended incision line, if the procedure is being done under local anesthesia, using 25 G 1-inch needle.
3. Feel the cord.
4. Attach and insert a 21 G 1.5-inch needle lateral to the cord and aspirate.
5. If no blood aspirated, inject around the cord, including the medial aspect.
6. Make sure to aspirate before injecting, every time you change position of the needle.

Penile Block

1. Withdraw your local anesthetic into a 20-mL syringe using a 21 G 1.5-inch needle, then dispose of the needle accordingly.
2. Palpate the symphysis pubis at the level of the base of the penis.
3. Attach and insert a 23 G (0.64-mm outer diameter) 1.5-inch long needle, through the skin, just below the symphysis pubis, until you reach the inferior border of the symphysis.
4. Advance the needle by 1–2 cm until you feel a loss of resistance.
5. At that stage you would have entered through the superficial fascia of the penis and into Buck's fascia.
6. Aspirate for blood. If no blood aspirated, inject approximately one-half the local anesthetic to block the dorsal nerve.
7. Withdraw the needle slightly and maneuver it to one side of the penis and then to the other side. Be careful to avoid the dorsal artery of the penis as you are moving the needle from one side to the other.
8. Inject approximately one-half of the remaining local anesthetic on both sides of the penis. This will block the ilioinguinal and genitofemoral nerves.
9. Sometimes, this block does not offer full anesthesia in the area of the distal ventral aspect of the penis around the frenulum and you may need to inject anesthetic locally in that area as you make your incisions there (one-quarter of the local anesthetic should be reserved for this maneuver).

References

1. Norris RL Jr. Local Anesthetics. Emerg Med Clin North Am. 1992;10(4):707–18.
2. Catterall W, Mackie K. Local Anesthetics. In: Hardman JG, Limbird LE, Gilman AG, eds. *The Pharmacological Basis of Therapeutics*. 10th ed. New York: McGraw-Hill, 2001:367–84.

6. Reduction of Torsion of Testis and Fixation

Hashim Hashim and Paul Abrams

Indications

Testicular torsion is a surgical emergency and should be operated on immediately once a diagnosis is made. The patient should be consented for reduction of torsion, bilateral testicular fixation, orchidectomy (if needed), and insertion of testicular prosthesis (if needed).

Procedure: Simple Orchidectomy

1. The operation is normally performed under general/regional anesthesia.
2. Ask the anesthetist to give intravenous antibiotics at induction (e.g., third-generation cephalosporin).
3. Place the patient in the supine position.
4. Shave the scrotum and prepare the lower abdomen, penis, and scrotum with aqueous betadine or chlorhexidine. Drape accordingly.
5. Pull the testis down to relax the cremaster.
6. Grasp the scrotum around and behind the torted testis with the fingers and thumb of one hand and compress the testis against the anterior scrotal wall to stretch the skin over it (Figure 6.1).
7. One of two incisions can be made (Figure 6.2). They only need to be approximately 3–5 cm long:
   - Unilateral transverse incision within the scrotal folds and between the scrotal vessels
   - Median raphe incision. This is our preferred incision, as it allows good access to both testes and results in minimal bleeding with a good postoperative scar.
8. Once the skin is incised, keep the testis under compression and incise the dartos muscle and the underlying cremasteric layers one by one from one edge of the wound to the other. Stop when you reach the tunica vaginalis, which may appear darkened owing to to an acute bloody hydrocele. Control any bleeding with bipolar diathermy.

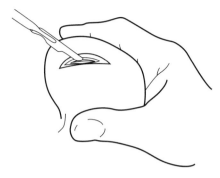

Figure 6.1. Grasping the Scrotum.

9. Push all the scrotal layers away from the testis using a swab. The testis can at this stage be delivered with the tunica vaginalis and then the tunica vaginalis incised. Alternatively, the tunica vaginalis can be opened while the testis is still in the scrotum and then the testis delivered. Drain any hydrocele fluid.
10. A diagnosis of torsion is made if the cord is twisted.
11. Observe the color of the testis before detorsion then untwist the testis:
12. Cover the affected testis with warm saline-soaked swabs and wait for 5–10 minutes.
13. In the meantime, explore the contralateral side either through the same incision if using a midline incision or make another incision on the contralateral side if using a transverse incision.

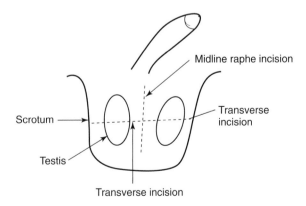

Figure 6.2. Scrotal Incisions.

14. Deliver the contralateral testis, evert the edges of the tunica vaginalis, and place a few interrupted 3/0 synthetic absorbable sutures to approximate the edges behind the testis (*see* Chapter 11; Jaboulay procedure). There is no evidence that this reduces the risk of subsequent torsion; however, the aim is to reduce the risk of hydrocele formation.

15. Fix the contralateral testis. There is controversy as to whether fixation should be with absorbable or non-absorbable material. The advantage of using absorbable sutures is that they dissolve and therefore the stitches cannot be felt later through the scrotum. However, there is a theoretical risk that the chance of a recurrent torsion is higher. The advantage of the non-absorbable sutures is that they do not dissolve, and the risk of torsion is theoretically lower; however, the stitches can sometimes be felt through the scrotal skin. Our preference is to use 4/0 monofilament absorbable suture, as this takes longer to dissolve than the braided absorbable sutures, slides easier through the testis, and thus causes less trauma than a braided suture. The risk of recurrent torsion with absorbable stitches is probably extremely low and only theoretical, as the testis will be held in place by the inflammatory tissue reaction around the stitches, resulting in fibrous fixation.

16. The testis is fixed in a three-point fixation by inserting two stitches through the tunica albuginea, one stitch on the medial aspect of the testis, and one stitch on the lateral aspect of the testis, near the superior pole of the testis. Try to avoid the anterior wall of the testis, as it is vascular. A third stitch can be placed on the medial or lateral side lower than the other stitches (Figure 6.3). Do not tie the stitches at this stage. The stitches can also be placed all on one side, either medial or lateral.

17. Invert the scrotal skin into the wound using the finger of your hand and pass the three sutures at appropriate positions into the dartos muscle so that the testis can lie in its natural position.

18. Push the testis back into the scrotum and tie the sutures at this stage.

19. Now go back and inspect the torted testis:
    - If the color has changed back to normal, then follow points 15–18 above.
    - If the color is not back to normal, then make a small incision in the tunica albuginea.

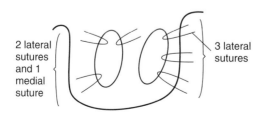

Figure 6.3. Placement of Sutures When Fixing the Testis.

- If the color of the seminiferous tubules is dark and no bright red bleeding occurs (arterial) with only dark venous blood then it is probably not viable and orchidectomy must be considered (*see* Chapter 7). Consider placing a prosthesis (*see* Chapter 9) at the same time as orchidectomy, using the same incision. If there is any doubt about viability, then it is probably better to leave the testis in position.
- If bright red arterial bleeding is observed, then the testis may well regain its function and normal color once it is inside the scrotum and the testis should be salvaged and fixed with the three-point technique as described previously. You will need to follow the patient up with Doppler ultrasound scanning in approximately 1 week to make sure that there is flow to the testis. If there is no flow, then a simple orchidectomy may need to be considered, especially if there is pain or signs of sepsis.

20. Some surgeons advocate placing the testis in a dartos pouch rather than back into its normal position to reduce the risk of recurrent torsion. A dartos pouch can be developed digitally between the dartos and external spermatic fascia. The testis is then fixed in the pouch using three-point fixation as well.

21. Close the dartos muscle with undyed 3/0 synthetic absorbable suture in a continuous fashion.

22. Inject 0.5% marcaine into the skin edges and dartos to reduce the post-operative pain.

23. Close the skin with interrupted undyed 4/0 synthetic absorbable suture to avoid staining of the skin. Alternatively, you can use surgical glue or use a subcuticular monofilament continuous suture.

24. Cover the wound with non-stick dressing.

25. Give the patient a scrotal support to reduce post-operative hematoma.

26. The patient can normally go home the same day.

27. If no torsion or evidence of any other pathology, such as epididymo-orchitis, is found at Step 10 above, then the testis should still be fixed and returned to its normal position, as it may have twisted and then untwisted. Fixing the other testis is debatable in this situation. But if a decision was made not to fix the other testis, it should be clearly explained to the patient that the other testis was not fixed and he may have similar symptoms in the future and may require further exploration.

28. If, at Step 10, a torted hydatid of Morgagni is found rather than a torted testis, then the testis is also NOT fixed but the hydatid is removed by either ligating its base with 4/0 synthetic absorbable suture or electro-cauterizing it and then cutting it.

Complications

Occasional complications include:

- Infection of the wound, requiring further treatment with antibiotics or surgery

- Bleeding from the wound and formation of scrotal hematoma, requiring surgery
- Feeling the stitch used to fix the testis

Rare complications include:

- Retorsion
- Loss of fertility in future
- Loss of testicular size or atrophy in future if testis is saved
- Remote possibility that an unsuspected diagnosis may be found on the histology examination, requiring further treatment

References

1. Reduction of testis torsion. In: *Atlas of Urologic Surgery, 2nd Edition*. Hinman F Jr (Ed). Philadelphia: Saunders; 1998;347–348.
2. The British Association of Urological Surgeons (Consent forms). http://www.baus. org.uk. Date accessed: May 25, 2007.
3. Pearce I, Islam S, McIntyre IG, O'Flynn KJ. Suspected testicular torsion: a survey of clinical practice in North West England. J R Soc Med 2002;95:247–249.

7. Simple and Subcapsular Orchidectomies (Orchiectomies)

Hashim Hashim and Paul Abrams

Indications

Orchidectomy is the removal of a testis. It may be simple or radical. The indications for simple orchidectomy are:

- Unsalvageable testicular trauma
- Severe recurrent or chronic testicular pain
- Testicular infarction (e.g., following testicular torsion)
- Part of gender reassignment surgery
- Management of prostatic carcinoma (subcapsular orchidectomy)

Procedure: Simple Orchidectomy

Simple orchidectomies are usually performed through a scrotal skin incision, but can be performed via a groin incision.

1. The most important action, before the operation, is to mark the correct operative side (i.e., right or left) and to include that in the consent form.
2. The possibility of insertion of a prosthesis should also be discussed with the patient.
3. The operation is normally performed under general/regional anesthesia.
4. Ask the anesthetist to give intravenous antibiotics at induction (e.g., third-generation cephalosporin).
5. Place the patient in the supine position.
6. Shave the scrotum and prepare the lower abdomen, penis, and scrotum with aqueous betadine or chlorhexidine. Drape accordingly.
7. Pull the testis down to relax the cremaster.
8. Grasp the scrotum around and behind the testis with the fingers and thumb of one hand and compress the testis against the anterior scrotal wall to stretch the skin over it (*see* Figure 6.1).
9. One of two incisions can be made (*see* Figure 6.2). They only need to be approximately 3–5 cm:

- Unilateral transverse incision within the scrotal folds and between the scrotal vessels
- Median raphe incision. This is our preferred incision, as it allows good access to both testis and results in minimal bleeding with a good postoperative scar.

10. Once the skin is incised, keep the testis under compression and incise the dartos muscle and the underlying cremasteric layers one by one from one edge of the wound to the other. Stop when you reach the bluish tunica vaginalis. Control any bleeding with bipolar diathermy.

11. Push all the scrotal layers away from the testis using a swab. The testis can at this stage be delivered with the tunica vaginalis and then the tunica vaginalis incised. Alternatively, the tunical vaginalis can be opened while the testis is still in the scrotum and then the testis is delivered.

12. Gently pull the testis down to expose the epididymis and cord.

13. Make sure there is no hernia in the cord. If there is a lipoma, then excise it.

14. You can put a clamp across the whole cord, but it can be thick and difficult to ligate. Therefore it is better to separate the cord into two or three parts.

15. Gently and bluntly, using tissue scissors, separate the spermatic vessels from the vas deferens. The vas normally lies anterior and the vessels posterior to it.

16. Place two clamps proximally (cranially), one above the other with approximately 1 cm between them on the vas, and one distal approximately 2 cm from the lower of the two proximal clamps.

17. Divide the vas between the distal and proximal clamps using tissue scissors. Ligate the vas below the distal clamp and remove the clamp. Then ligate the vas above the lower proximal clamp and remove it, and then ligate above the top proximal clamp and remove the clamp. 3/0 synthetic absorbable sutures can be used for ligation.

18. Repeat Steps 13 and 14 over the other part of the cord that includes the vessels.

19. The advantage of placing two proximal clamps and ligating the proximal (cranial) part of the cord twice is to avoid loss of the vessels, as they can retract very quickly and can cause a hematoma if not ligated properly. Alternatively, you can suture-ligate the vessels, with a trans-fixing stitch.

20. Place the testis in a kidney dish and hand it over to the scrub nurse.

21. Ensure that hemostasis is achieved before closure.

22. At this stage a prosthesis can be inserted (*see* Chapter 9 on insertion of prosthesis).

23. If there is infection or you are worried about bleeding, then a corrugated drain can be inserted, coming out through the most dependent part of the scrotum and fixed in place with a 2/0 non-absorbable suture and safety pin.

24. Close the dartos muscle with undyed 3/0 absorbable suture in a continuous fashion.

25. Inject 0.5% marcaine into the skin edges and dartos to reduce the post-operative pain.
26. Close the skin with interrupted undyed 4/0 synthetic absorbable suture to avoid staining of the skin. Alternatively, you can use surgical glue or use a subcuticular monofilament continuous suture.
27. Cover the wound with a non-stick dressing.
28. Give the patient a scrotal support to reduce post-operative hematoma.
29. The patient can normally go home the same day.

Procedure: Subcapsular (Intracapsular) Orchidectomy

1. Usually bilateral in the management of prostate cancer
2. Follow Steps 1 to 12 in the previous section.
3. Once the testis is delivered, incise the tunica albuginea of the testis along its length.
4. Clamp the sides of the tunica albuginea with two or three clamps on each side and evert the edges.
5. Using a gauze swab, use the index finger to swipe off all the tubules from the inner layer of the tunica albuginea. This tends to bleed and you will need to electrocauterize the bleeding vessels as they appear.
6. The tubules will be attached to the hilum inside the tunica albuginea. Clamp, ligate, and divide the hilus and electrocauterize it to stop any bleeding (Figure 7.1).
7. Electrocauterize all the internal surface of the tunica albuginea to destroy any residual cells that may produce testosterone.
8. Suture the edges of the tunica albuginea with a continuous 3/0 synthetic absorbable suture.
9. Replace the testis back into the scrotum.
10. Ensure that hemostasis is achieved before closure.
11. Close the dartos muscle with undyed 3/0 absorbable suture in a continuous fashion.
12. Open the contralateral hemiscrotum through the same midline incision and deliver the testis as before. Follow the previous steps.

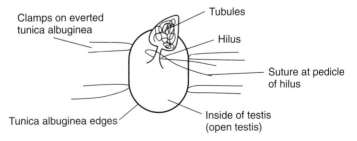

Figure 7.1. Removing the Hilus in a Subcapsular Orchidectomy.

13. Inject 0.5% marcaine into the skin edges and dartos to reduce the post-operative pain.
14. Close the skin with interrupted undyed 4/0 synthetic absorbable suture to avoid staining of the skin. Alternatively, you can use surgical glue or use a subcuticular monofilament continuous suture.
15. Cover the wound with non-stick dressing.
16. Give the patient scrotal support to reduce post-operative hematoma.
17. The patient can normally go home the same day.

Complications

Occasional complications include:

- Infection of the wound, requiring further treatment with antibiotics or surgery
- Bleeding from the wound and formation of scrotal hematoma, requiring surgery
- Potential loss of fertility

Rare complications include:

- Finding of an unsuspected diagnosis on the histology examination, requiring further treatment
- Remote possibility that the pathological diagnosis will be uncertain

References

1. Simple orchiectomy. In: *Atlas of Urologic Surgery, 2nd Edition.* Hinman F Jr (Ed), Philadelphia: Saunders; 1998; 375–378.
2. The British Association of Urological Surgeons (Consent forms). http://www.baus.org.uk. Date accessed: May 25, 2007.

8. Radical Orchidectomy (Orchiectomy)

Hashim Hashim and Paul Abrams

Indications

Orchidectomy is the removal of a testis. It may be simple or radical. The main indication for radical orchidectomy is the presence of testicular cancer. It involves removal of the entire cord and testis.

Procedure

Radical orchidectomies are performed through a groin/inguinal incision.

1. The most important action, before the operation, is to mark the correct operative side (i.e., right or left) and to include that in the consent form.
2. The possibility of insertion of a prosthesis should also be discussed with the patient.
3. Permission to biopsy the other testis if small, abnormal, or if there is a history of maldescent should be sought.
4. The operation is normally performed under general/regional anesthesia.
5. Place the patient in the supine position.
6. Shave the scrotum and lower abdomen and prepare the lower abdomen, penis, and scrotum with aqueous betadine or chlorhexidine. Drape accordingly.
7. Make an incision in the skin, on the appropriate side, starting 2 cm above the pubic tubercle and extending approximately 5–7 cm parallel to the inguinal ligament to expose the external inguinal ring. This incision can be extended into the upper scrotum for large tumors.
8. Incise subcutaneous fat, Camper's fascia, and Scarpa's fascia. Any veins encountered during this step should either be clamped, divided, and ligated with 3/0 synthetic absorbable suture, or electrocauterized with diathermy.
9. Place a self-retaining retractor to open the wound.
10. Identify the external inguinal ring and the fibers of the external oblique. Incise the external oblique along its fibers starting from the external ring.
11. Beware of the ilioinguinal nerve, which lies just beneath the external oblique fascia. You need to identify and mobilize it so as not to resect it during the orchidectomy.
12. Grasp both edges of the external oblique with clamps.
13. Bluntly dissect the spermatic cord to expose the pubic tubercle. This can be done with peanut dissectors and by sweeping the index finger gently along the pubic tubercle so that the index finger can be placed under and around the cord.

14. Now lift the cord and free it all the way to the internal inguinal ring (1–2 cm above the midpoint of the inguinal ligament). Make sure there is no hernia in the cord.
15. Double clamp the cord at the internal inguinal ring, leaving about 1 cm between the two clamps (Figure 8.1).
16. Pull the testis out of the scrotum by pulling the cord near the pubic tubercle and also applying upward pressure on the scrotum under the testis. If the tumor is large, you can extend the incision over the antero-lateral aspect of the scrotum.
17. The testis is attached to the scrotum by the gubernaculum. This can either be electrocauterized or clamped, divided, and ligated. Be careful not to cause a hole in the scrotum while doing this maneuver.
18. Deliver the testis into the operating field. Place a clamp 1 cm below the two other clamps and divide between this clamp and the other two clamps. You should have a clamp on the specimen side and two clamps on the patient side (Figure 8.2).
19. Place the testis in a specimen dish and send for pathology.
20. Suture ligate the cord on the patient's side with 1/0 synthetic absorbable suture below the clamp nearer the internal inguinal ring and remove the clamp (Figure 8.3). Leave the length of the suture long (4–5 cm) to allow easy identification.
21. Suture ligate the cord with 1/0 synthetic absorbable suture on a needle below the other clamp and then remove the clamp (Figure 8.4). You can electrocoagulate the end of the cord on the patient's side at this stage.
22. Irrigate the wound, including the scrotum, with saline and ensure that hemostasis is maintained before closure.
23. It is at this stage that a prosthesis can be inserted (*see* Chapter 9).
24. Close the external oblique fascia and external ring in a continuous running fashion using 3/0 synthetic absorbable suture.

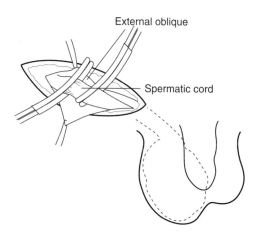

External oblique

Spermatic cord

Figure 8.1. Clamping the Cord at the Internal Ring.

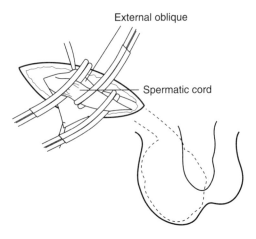

Figure 8.2. Placing a Third Clamp 1 cm Below the Other Two Clamps.

25. Appose Scarpa's fascia in an interrupted fashion using 3/0 synthetic absorbable suture.
26. Inject 0.5% marcaine into the skin edges and fascia and along the ilioinguinal nerve to reduce the post-operative pain.
27. Close the skin with subcuticular 3/0 monofilament absorbable continuous suture. Alternatively, you can use surgical glue or skin clips (need to be removed in 10 days post-operatively).
28. Cover the wound with a dressing of your choice.
29. Give the patient scrotal support to reduce post-operative hematoma.

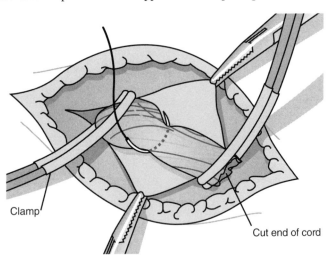

Figure 8.3. Suture Ligate Below the Most Proximal Clamp.

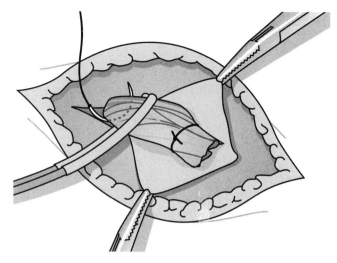

Figure 8.4. Placing a Suture Below the remaining Clamp.

30. The patient can normally go home the same day and resume routine daily activities in approximately 1–2 weeks.
31. Arrange appropriate follow-up.

Complications

Occasional complications include:

- Bleeding resulting in a hematoma or retroperitoneal bleeding may require further surgery to stop the bleeding
- Injury to the ilioinguinal nerve, resulting in loss of sensation to the ipsilateral groin and lateral hemiscrotum
- Infection of incision, requiring further treatment with antibiotics
- Cancer, if found, may require further treatment with procedures such as radiation or chemotherapy

Rare complications include:

- Removal of testes only to find that cancer was not present
- Loss of future fertility

References

1. Radical orchiectomy. In: *Atlas of Urologic Surgery, 2nd Edition*. Hinman F Jr (Ed), Philadelphia: Saunders; 1998; 380–384.
2. The British Association of Urological Surgeons (Consent forms). http://www.baus. org.uk. Date accessed: 5/25/07.

9. Insertion of Testicular Prosthesis (Implant)

Hashim Hashim and Paul Abrams

Indications

Testicular prostheses are inserted in patients who have a missing testicle, mainly for cosmetic and/or psychological reasons, and usually after removal of a testis for maldescent or tumor. The main contra-indications for insertion of a testicular implant are untreated cancer or the presence of infection. The two main types of prostheses available are ones that are filled with either silicone or saline.

The Mentor saline prosthesis (Figure 9.1) comes in four sizes. The implant is made of a molded silicone elastomer shell that is approximately 0.035-inches thick. It is not visible on X-ray. The device is filled with saline at the time of surgery and just prior to implantation. It includes a self-sealing injection site at one end, which allows for filling with a sterile saline solution. On the opposite end of the implant is a silicone elastomer tab, which enables suturing and securing the implant in a set position.

The Silimed highly polymerized silicone prosthesis (Figure 9.2) also comes in four sizes. It is composed of an envelope made of chemically and mechanically resistant silicone elastomer. It comes pre-filled with silicone and has a cap, which allows placement of the suture on one side. Dimensions of the two prosthesis types are compared in Table 9.1.

Procedure

A prosthesis can be inserted at the same time as an inguinoscrotal surgical procedure or at a later stage. It is easier if done at the same time because when the original testis is removed, it can be sutured to the gubernacular remnant and fit naturally in the position of the removed testicle. However, if there is a delay after the original surgery, then significant scarring and contraction of the scrotum develops, which can cause some difficulty in placing the prosthesis. We will describe the procedure for late implantation here.

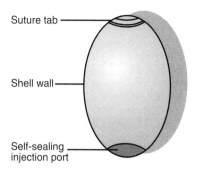

Figure 9.1. Saline-Filled Testicular Implants.

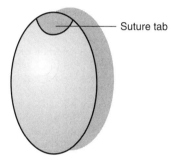

Figure 9.2. Silicone-Filled Testicular Implant.

1. The most important action, before the operation, is to mark the correct operative side (i.e., right or left) and to include that in the consent form.
2. The operation is normally performed under general/regional anesthesia.
3. Choose the appropriate size of prosthesis based on the size of the contralateral testis.

Table 9.1. Dimensions of the Two Prosthesis Types.

	Silimed (silicone-filled)		Mentor (saline-filled)	
	Length (cm)	Width (cm)	Length (cm)	Width (cm)
Extra-small	2.3	2.0	3.0	2.2
Small	3.4	2.5	3.5	2.5
Medium	4.2	3.0	4.0	2.7
Large	4.7	3.2	4.5	2.9

4. Place the patient in the supine position.
5. Shave the scrotum and lower abdomen and prepare the lower abdomen, penis, and scrotum with aqueous betadine or chlorhexidine. Drape accordingly.
6. Make an incision in the skin, on the appropriate side, starting 2 cm above the pubic tubercle and extending approximately 5–7 cm parallel to the inguinal ligament (same incision as for hernia repair) to expose the external inguinal ring. You can go through the old scar if the patient had an inguinal orchidectomy.
7. Alternatively, a scrotal median raphe incision can be made; however, if a prosthesis is being placed with this incision, then there is risk of necrosis to the skin and possibility of incising through the posterior wall of the scrotum. Therefore this incision should not be the first choice and used in only certain circumstances.
8. Incise subcutaneaous fat, Camper's fascia, and Scarpa's fascia. Any veins encountered during this step should either be clamped, divided and ligated with 3/0 synthetic absorbable suture, or electrocauterized with diathermy.
9. Place a self-retaining retractor to open the wound.
10. Identify the external inguinal ring and the fibers of the external oblique. Incise the external oblique along its fibers starting from the external ring.
11. Beware of the ilioinguinal nerve, which lies just beneath the external oblique fascia. You need to identify and mobilize it so as not to divide it during the procedure. The position may have changed if there has been previous surgery through that incision.
12. Grasp both edges of the external oblique with clamps to help expose the surgical field.
13. Use your fingers to identify the neck and previous tunnel to the scrotum. This usually commences at the external ring.
14. Pass your finger into the neck of the scrotum, to identify the path through which the prosthesis is going to be inserted and divide any adhesions. The aim is to create a pouch in which the prosthesis can sit. Be careful not to stretch the scrotal neck, as this can cause migration of the prosthesis.
15. Gently advance a pair of standard Rampley sponge-holding forceps through the scrotal neck down into the scrotum. The fulcrum of the forceps is positioned to align with the scrotal neck so the neck is not stretched. Any further dense adhesions or existing prosthesis capsule (from a previously inserted prosthesis) are divided and fractured by opening and closing the forceps in a gentle spreading motion. When closed, the forceps tips approximate the position of the prosthesis, indicating if further dissection is necessary.
16. An alternative to Step 15 above is to insert a 16-F Foley catheter with a 30-mL balloon into the scrotum. The balloon is initially inflated with 10 mL of water and positioned satisfactorily in the most dependant part of the scrotum. The balloon is inflated until its volume is similar to that of the contralateral testicle, and the volume recorded. A small

prosthesis equates to a catheter balloon volume of 18 mL, medium to 24 mL, and large to 30 mL. Deflate the balloon before removing the catheter.

17. Irrigate the wound, including the scrotum, with saline or an iodine-based antiseptic and ensure that hemostasis is maintained.
18. Either use your finger or a narrow tissue holding forceps, placed on the scrotal skin from the outside at its most dependant position, and push cranially upwards towards the direction of the inguinal wound to invert the scrotal skin.
19. Secure the prosthesis via its tab to the dartos layer at base of the scrotum, at the site marked by the finger or the Allis, using a 3/0 synthetic absorbable or non-absorbable suture. Be careful not to puncture the implant. Some surgeons prefer not to leave the prosthesis via its tab and just place it in the scrotum then close the scrotal neck with absorbable suture to stop the prosthesis from migrating into the inguinal region.
20. Gently push the prosthesis down into the pouch created in the scrotum and then "milk down" the scrotal skin and prosthesis from the outside to confirm satisfactory position.
21. Close the external oblique fascia and external ring in a continuous running fashion using 3/0 synthetic absorbable suture.
22. The wound is closed in layers and Scarpa's fascia is closed in an interrupted fashion using 3/0 synthetic absorbable suture.
23. Inject 0.5% marcaine into the skin edges and fascia and along the ilioinguinal nerve to reduce post-operative pain.
24. Close the skin with subcuticular 3/0 monofilament absorbable continuous suture. Alternatively, you can use surgical glue or skin clips (need to be removed in 10 days post-operatively).
25. Cover the wound with a dressing of your choice.
26. Give the patient scrotal support to go home with.
27. After surgery the patients are encouraged to "milk down" the prosthesis to maintain it in the pouch region until healed and a peri-prosthetic fibrous pseudo-capsule has developed.
28. The patient can normally go home the same day and resume routine activities, including intercourse, after approximately 1 week.

Complications

Occasional complications include:

- Pain, infection, or leaking, requiring removal of prosthesis
- Cosmetic result is not always perfect, especially in terms of size
- Prosthesis may become displaced, migrate, or extrude
- Palpable stitch at one end, which you may be able to feel if a non-absorbable suture is used. An abscess may also form around the stitch that may need surgical treatment

- Scar tissue (capsule) around the testicular implant may contract, causing fibrous capsular contracture and resulting in pain
- The long-term risks from use of silicone products is unknown
- Hematoma formation caused by bleeding from the inside of the scrotum
- The length of time the implant can stay *in situ* is unknown and may need replacement in the future.

References

1. Coloplast – Testicular Implants. http://www.urology.coloplast.com/. Date accessed: May 25, 2007.
2. Polytech Silimed Europe GmbH. http://www.polytechsilimed.info. Date accessed: May 25, 2007.
3. Simms MS, Huq S, Mellon JK. Testicular prostheses: a new technique for insertion. BJU Int 2004;93(1):179.
4. Lawrentschuk N, Webb D. Inserting testicular prostheses: a new surgical technique for difficult cases. BJU Int 2005;95(7):1111–1114.
5. The British Association of Urological Surgeons (Consent forms). http://www.baus.org.uk. Date accessed: May 25, 2007.

10. Testicular Biopsy

Hashim Hashim and Paul Abrams

Indications

Testicular biopsy is the removal of a small piece of testicular tissue through a scrotal incision. It can be performed using ultrasound with a needle, but this has some disadvantages (discussed later). It is usually performed to help determine the cause of male infertility when the man has an abnormal sperm count (azoospermia) and normal leutenizing (LH) and follicle-stimulating (FSH) hormones. The findings help distinguish between testicular failure and post-testicular causes of infertility.

Procedure

1. The operation is normally performed under general/regional anesthesia, but can be performed under local anesthesia.
2. Place the patient in the supine position.
3. Shave the scrotum and prepare the penis and scrotum with aqueous betadine or chlorhexidine. Drape accordingly.
4. Pull the testis, which may be small, down to relax the cremaster.
5. Grasp the scrotum around and behind the testis with the fingers and thumb of one hand and compress the testis against the anterior scrotal wall to stretch the skin over it (*see* Figure 6.1).
6. One of two incisions can be made (*see* Figure 6.2). They only need to be approximately 3–5 cm long:
   - Unilateral transverse incision within the scrotal folds and between the scrotal vessels.
   - Median raphe incision. This is our preferred incision, as it allows good access to both testis and results in minimal bleeding with a good post-operative scar.
7. Once the skin is incised, keep the testis under compression and incise the dartos muscle and the underlying cremasteric layers one by one from one edge of the wound to the other. Stop when you reach the bluish tunica vaginalis. Control any bleeding with bipolar diathermy.
8. Push all the scrotal layers away from the testis using a swab. The testis can at this stage be delivered within the tunica vaginalis and then the

tunica vaginalis incised. Alternatively, the tunica vaginalis can be opened while the testis is still in the scrotum and then the testis is delivered.

9. Make a small 3- to 5-mm transverse incision in the tunica albuginea in the superior medial or lateral aspect of the testicle. The anterior part is more vascular. Testicular seminiferous tubules should start to extrude. If they don't, then give the testicle a small squeeze. But be careful, as a lot of tubules can come out. Do not squeeze the testis hard.

10. Excise a small amount of extruded tubules with tissue scissors and send it to the laboratory in buffered glutaraldehyde solution.

11. Push the rest of the tubules back into the testis.

12. Close the tunica albuginea with one or two interrupted 4/0 synthetic absorbable sutures.

13. Maintain hemostasis. You may need to add more sutures to stop the bleeding.

14. Evert the tunica vaginalis to prevent formation of a hydrocele and approximate the edges with two or three interrupted 3/0 synthetic absorbable sutures.

15. Close the dartos muscle with undyed 3/0 absorbable suture in a continuous fashion.

16. Repeat the procedure on the opposite side, if indicated.

17. Inject 0.5% bupivicaine hydrochloride (marcaine) into the skin edges and dartos to reduce the post-operative pain.

18. Close the skin with interrupted undyed 4/0 synthetic absorbable suture to avoid staining of the skin. Alternatively, you can use surgical glue or use a subcuticular monofilament continuous suture.

19. Cover the wound with non-adhesive dressing.

20. Give the patient a scrotal support to help reduce post-operative hematoma.

21. The patient can normally go home the same day.

Testicular biopsies can be performed using percutaneous needles and under ultrasound guidance; however, the main disadvantages of this technique are that a testicular blood vessel may be inadvertently damaged without being recognized, only small amounts of tissue are obtained for histology, and distortion of the tubules may make histological interpretation difficult.

Complications

Occasional complications include:

- Bleeding, requiring further treatment such as antibiotics or surgery
- Inconclusive diagnosis from biopsy

Rare complications include:

- Damage to the testicle, epididymis, or vas deferens from biopsy
- Chronic pain in the testicle or scrotum
- Potential loss of fertility in the future

References

1. Testis biopsy. In: *Atlas of Urologic Surgery, 2nd Edition.* Hinman F Jr (Ed). Philadelphia: Saunders; 1998; 305–307.
2. The British Association of Urological Surgeons (Consent forms). http://www.baus.org.uk. Date accessed: May 25, 2007.

11. Hydrocele Repair in Adults

Hashim Hashim and Paul Abrams

Indications

A hydrocele is an accumulation of fluid within the tunica vaginalis. Hydroceles are usually painless, but can cause discomfort because of their size. The main indication for operating would be a symptomatic troublesome swelling that has an effect on quality of life (e.g., difficulty in wearing trousers). Hydrocele repair is the removal or repair of the fluid sac surrounding the testicle. This is normally done through a scrotal incision.

A scrotal ultrasound scan should be performed before doing a hydrocele repair to look for any intratesticular pathology. Should there be any pathology then an inguinal approach is indicated. If there is an inguinoscrotal hernia, then the inguinal approach is also indicated.

Procedure

1. The operation is normally performed under general/regional anesthesia. It can be performed under local anesthesia using a cord block, but can be painful.
2. Place the patient in the supine position share the scrotum and prepare the lower abdomen and scrotum with aqueous betadine. Drape accordingly.
3. Pull the testis down to relax the cremaster.
4. Grasp the scrotum with one hand and compress the hydrocele against the anterior scrotal wall to stretch the skin over the hydrocele.
5. One of two incisions can be made (*see* Chapter 6). They only need to be approximately 3 cm:
   - Transverse incision within the scrotal folds and between the scrotal vessels.
   - Median raphe incision. This is our preferred incision, as it allows good access to both testes and results in minimal bleeding with a good post-operative scar.
6. Once the skin is incised, keep the hydrocele under compression and incise the dartos muscle and the underlying layers one by one from one edge of the wound to the other. Any bleeding should be controlled by bipolar diathermy.

7. Once you reach the tunica vaginalis, use your index finger to dissect the tunica vaginalis from the dartos in the avascular plane, as much as you can to free the sac. Then make a small stab incision. Be careful as the fluid may flow out under pressure and spray you or your assistant. To avoid this "fountaining" of fluid, place two pairs of Allis forceps on the tunica and incise between them.

8. Allow all the fluid to drain from the hydrocele into a receiver such as a kidney dish. Alternatively, you can use suction draining.

9. Once the fluid is drained, incise the tunica with dissecting scissors and deliver the testis outside the scrotum. Remove the Allis forceps.

10. Inspect and palpate the testis and epididymis. Make sure you identify the epididymis, vas deferens, and internal spermatic vessels to avoid damage to them.

11. Control any bleeding on the edges of the tunica with diathermy or oversaw with a 4/0 synthetic absorbable suture.

12. If the sac wall (tunica) is thick or the hydrocele is multi-loculated or very large, then excise the sac leaving about one-fingerbreadth margin to avoid injury to the epididymis. Evert the sac inside out and saw the free edges of the sac together behind the testis, leaving approximately 1 cm between the two edges (Jaboulay procedure, Figure 11.1). Use 3/0 synthetic absorbable continuous stitch on a curved needle. This reduces the chance of recurrence caused by re-apposition of the edges of the hydrocele sac and avoids strangulating the cord.

13. If the sac wall is thin, then you can plicate the sac edges (Lord's procedure, Figure 11.2). This is done by using 4/0 interrupted synthetic absorbable stitches. Insert the needle at the free edge of the sac and then pick up a small bite of the sac radially every 1 cm to gather up the sac wall until you reach the tunica albuginea of the testis. Now tie the suture. Repeat this suturing at regular intervals around the testis placing approximately 8–10 sutures in total.

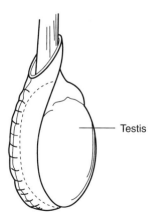

Testis

Figure 11.1. Jaboulay Procedure.

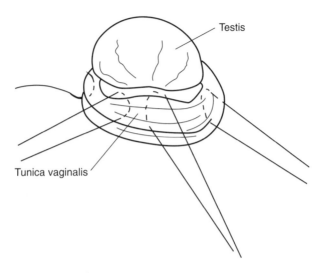

Figure 11.2. Lord's Procedure.

14. Ensure that hemostasis is maintained.
15. Pick up the cremaster (but not the skin) with two pairs of Allis forceps and return the testis into the scrotum. This may require some pressure. Make sure that it is in its natural and proper orientation and that you do not rotate it and cause a torsion.
16. You can do a cord block with 0.5% marcaine to reduce the post-operative pain before closing the dartos.
17. Close the dartos muscle with undyed 3/0 synthetic absorbable continuous suture.
18. Close the skin with interrupted undyed 4/0 synthetic absorbable suture to avoid staining of the skin. Alternatively, you can use surgical glue.
19. Give the patient scrotal support to reduce post-operative hematoma.
20. The patient can normally go home the same day.

In those patients who are not fit for an operation or who do not want an operation, drainage of the hydrocele can be done using a cannula, but the recurrence rate is high. This can be done in the following manner:

1. Place the patient in the supine position.
2. Darken the room slightly.
3. Shine a torch pen onto the scrotum to identify the hydrocele and the position of the testis.
4. Identify where the vessels are.
5. Clean the skin with an alcohol swab or aqueous betadine.
6. Inject some local anesthetic (e.g., 1% lidocaine) into the skin and deeper tissues.

7. Insert an 18 G intravenous cannula perpendicular to the anterior scrotal wall into the hydrocele, avoiding the scrotal wall vessels and the testis in the posterior aspect of the hydrocele.
8. Withdraw the needle but keep the cannula *in situ*.
9. Allow the fluid (yellow in color) to escape into a receiver, such as a kidney dish.
10. Squeeze the remaining fluid out until the sac is empty.
11. Aspirate the fluid with a syringe gradually to avoid any unnecessary damage to the testis, which may cause pain and bleeding.
12. A sclerosant can be instilled into the scrotum following aspiration. This includes sodium tetradecylsulphate, tetracycline, or polidocanol (aethoxysklerol).
13. Once finished, withdraw the cannula and pinch the puncture site for approximately 1 minute and cover it with a non-stick dressing.

Complications

Occasional complications include:

- Recurrence of the hydrocele. The excision technique seems to result in the lowest recurrence rate, but the highest complication rate.
- Hematoma formation, which normally resolves slowly but may require surgical drainage.
- Infection of the wound or the scrotal contents, requiring treatment with antibiotics. There is no difference in the rates of wound infection and hematoma formation between the two operative techniques.
- Scrotal edema.
- Damage to the epididymis and vas deferens, which can affect fertility and result in azoospermia when there is a single testis or the procedure is bilateral.

References

1. Kaye KW, Clayman RV, Lange PH. Outpatient hydrocele and spermatocele repair under local anesthesia. J Urol 1983;130:269.
2. Chalasani V, Woo HH. Why not use a small incision to treat large hydroceles? ANZ J Surg 2002;72:594.
3. Ku JH, Kim ME, Lee NK, Park YH. The excisional, plication and internal drainage techniques: a comparison of the results for idiopathic hydrocele. BJU Int 2001; 87:82.
4. Ross LS, Flom LS. Azoospermia: a complication of hydrocele repair in a fertile population. J Urol 1991;146:852.

5. Correction of hydrocele. In: *Atlas of Urologic Surgery, 2nd Edition*. Hinman F Jr (Ed). Philadelphia: Saunders; 1998; 349–351.

6. Daehlin L, Tonder B, Kapstad L. Comparison of polidocanol and tetracycline in the sclerotherapy of testicular hydrocele and epididymal cyst. Br J Urol 1997;80(3): 468–471.

7. Braslis KG, Moss DI. Long-term experience with sclerotherapy for treatment of epididymal cyst and hydrocele. Aust N Z J Surg 1996;66(4):222–224.

8. The British Association of Urological Surgeons (Consent forms). http://www.baus. org.uk. Date accessed: May 25, 2007.

12. Excision of Epididymal Cyst or Spermatocele

Hashim Hashim and Paul Abrams

Indications

This is an operation to remove a cyst attached to the epididymis, which in the case of the spermatocele contains sperm and in the case of an epididymal cyst, clear-/straw-colored fluid. The main indication for operating on an epididymal cyst is an increase in size of the cyst, causing discomfort or pain. Cysts rarely cause obstruction of the epididymis, but if they do and fertility is affected then removal of the cyst is another indication. Cysts may be single or multiple and some are multi-locular.

Procedure

1. The most important action, before the operation, is to mark the correct operative side (i.e., right or left) and to include that in the consent form.
2. The operation is normally performed under general/regional anesthesia.
3. Place the patient in the supine position.
4. Shave the scrotum and prepare the lower abdomen, penis, and scrotum with aqueous betadine or chlorhexidine. Drape accordingly.
5. Pull the testis down to relax the cremaster.
6. Grasp the scrotum around and behind the testis with the fingers and thumb of one hand and compress the testis against the anterior scrotal wall to stretch the skin over it (*see* Figure 6.1).
7. One of two incisions can be made (*see* Figure 6.2). They only need to be approximately 3–5 cm long, but can be bigger if the cyst is large:
    - Unilateral transverse incision, over the testis, within the scrotal folds and between the scrotal vessels. This is the preferred incision if the operation is unilateral.
    - Median raphe incision: allows good access to both testis and results in minimal bleeding with a good post-operative scar.
8. Once the skin is incised, keep the testis under compression and incise the dartos muscle and the underlying cremasteric layers one by one

from one edge of the wound to the other. Stop when you reach the tunica vaginalis. Control any bleeding with bipolar diathermy.

9. Push all the scrotal layers away from the testis using a swab. The testis can at this stage be delivered with the tunica vaginalis and then the tunica vaginalis incised. Alternatively, the tunica vaginalis can be opened while the testis is still in the scrotum and then the testis is delivered.
10. Gently pull the testis down to expose the epididymis and cord.
11. Begin cautious blunt and sharp dissection of the cyst with tissue scissors. Remove all the adventitial tissue of the cyst using gauze on a finger. The aim is to remove the cyst without puncturing it or damaging the epididymis and vessels. There will be bloodless tissue planes through which you will need to do the dissection.
12. If you inadvertently puncture the cyst, then place a mosquito clamp on the hole made in the cyst to stop the fluid from pouring out. It is difficult to dissect the whole cyst if there is no fluid left in it and thus it may recur later.
13. Proceed with dissection until you reach the base of the cyst, which is attached to the epididymis.
14. Clamp the base, then ligate and divide it on the epididymis side.
15. Close any defect in the epididymis with continuous 3/0 synthetic absorbable suture.
16. Ensure that hemostasis is achieved before closure.
17. Evert the tunica vaginalis behind the testis (*see* Chapter 11) to prevent formation of a hydrocele, and apply three or four interrupted 3/0 synthetic absorbable sutures to the tunica vaginalis.
18. Replace the testis in its natural position in the scrotum.
19. Close the dartos muscle with undyed 3/0 absorbable suture in a continuous fashion.
20. Inject 0.5% bupivicaine hydrochloride (marcaine) into the skin edges and dartos to reduce the post-operative pain.
21. Close the skin with interrupted undyed 4/0 synthetic absorbable suture to avoid staining of the skin. Alternatively, you can use surgical glue or use a subcuticular monofilament continuous suture.
22. Cover the wound with non-stick dressing.
23. Give the patient scrotal support to reduce post-operative hematoma.
24. The patient can normally go home the same day.

Complications

Occasional complications include:

- Recurrence of cyst
- Infection of the wound, requiring further treatment with antibiotics or surgery
- Bleeding from the wound and formation of scrotal hematoma, requiring surgery

Rare complications include:

- Future fertility could be affected because of scarring or damage to the epididymis

References

1. Spermatocelectomy. In: *Atlas of Urologic Surgery, 2nd Edition*. Hinman F Jr (Ed). Philadelphia: Saunders; 1998; 406–408.
2. The British Association of Urological Surgeons (Consent forms). http://www.baus. org.uk. Date accessed: May 25, 2007.

13. Vasectomy

Hashim Hashim and Paul Abrams

Indications

Vasectomy is an operation to cut or tie off the vas deferens, which carry sperm out of the testicles. The main indication is for sterilization as part of family planning, especially in couples who have the number of children they desire and in men whose wives cannot practice any other family planning methods, whether permanent or temporary. There are many techniques available; however, they all follow the same three principles of isolation of the vas deferens, delivery and interruption of the vas, and management of the vasal ends. We will explain the steps for the two most widely used techniques: scalpel and no-scalpel procedures.

Procedure: Scalpel Technique

This is normally performed under locally anesthesia; it is occasionally performed under general anesthesia, if one or other vas is difficult to feel (i.e., if there is a varicocele).

1. Apply topical local anesthetic (e.g., eutectic mixture of local anesthetics [EMLA] cream) to anesthetize the scrotal skin approximately 20–30 minutes before the procedure while the patient is waiting for the operation.
2. Place the patient in the supine position.
3. Shave the scrotum and remove the hair. It may be easier to stand on the patient's left side if you are right-handed and vice-versa, but the surgeon has to be comfortable with the position they choose.
4. Prepare the scrotal skin and penis with warm (to prevent scrotal contraction) aqueous povidone-iodine or chlorhexidine solution.
5. Drape accordingly and keep the penis away from the operative field.
6. Pull/retract the testis down to relax the cremaster with the non-dominant hand.
7. Isolating and securing the vas is probably the most challenging step. Use a "three-finger technique" for positioning the vas in which the non-dominant hand is used to manipulate and separate the vas away from the other cord structures and into a subcutaneous position

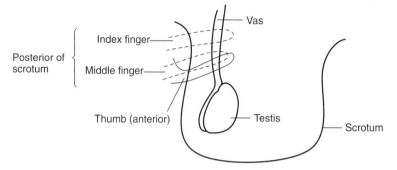

Figure 13.1. Holding the Vas in Place.

between the thumb anteriorly and the index and middle fingers posteriorly (Figure 13.1).

8. Make a 1- to 2-cm wheal at the desired incision site with 1% lidocaine without epinephrine, usually at the junction of the middle and upper one-third in the lateral part of the scrotum, bilaterally. A 50:50 mixture of 1% lidocaine and 0.5% bupivacaine is an alternative because of lidocaine's rapid onset of action and bupivacaine's longer-lasting anesthetic effect.

9. Advanced the needle through the wheal, without injecting the anesthetic, parallel and adjacent to the vas and toward the external inguinal ring to provide a vasal nerve block. After gentle aspiration, 2–5 mL of anesthetic is injected into the external spermatic fascia. Wait for approximately 3 minutes.

10. Make a 0.5- to 1-cm horizontal or vertical incision using a scalpel.

11. Place a ring-end clamp or towel clip around the vas so that it does not retract into the scrotum. Try not to place the clamp through the skin, as this can be painful.

12. Bluntly dissect the soft tissue around the vas with a fine curved hemostat.

13. The vas and surrounding tissue may then be elevated through the incision. Warn the patient that this may cause some pain and inject more lidocaine.

14. Compress the scrotum on either side around the vas between the thumb and index finger to thin the tissue overlying the vas.

15. Incise the fibrous layer surrounding the vas longitudinally until you reach the white wall of the vas.

16. Fully isolate the vas from the fibrous layers along a length of approximately 2–3 cm using the hemostat. It is important to keep the ring-end clamp or towel clip in position.

17. Apply two clamps on the vas: one distal to the towel clip and one proximal to the clip at least 15 mm apart (Figure 13.2).

18. Use a scissors or scalpel to remove at least 15 mm of vas. The removed segment may be sent for pathologic examination to confirm that the

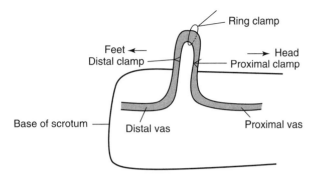

Figure 13.2. Placing the Clamps on the Vas.

vas has been removed rather than the artery (this adds unnecessary cost with little benefit, in experienced hands).

19. Different techniques exist for management of the two vasal ends and combination techniques are usually performed.

   - Ligation with 3/0 synthetic absorbable sutures: the vas is turned in a U-turn fashion and a suture is placed around the two arms of the U-shape (Figure 13.3). This can result in ischemic necrosis and sloughing of the vasal ends.
   - Clipping: Surgical clips can be felt through the scrotum and may cause discomfort. Sometimes they can become dislodged.
   - Luminal fulgration: Cautery should be inserted 3–4 mm into the cut ends and withdrawn slowly. It creates a third-degree burn, which subsequently produces a scar that seals the end. Thermal cautery seems to cause less vasitis nodosa (blind channels lined with epithelium arising from the lumen of the vas) and sperm granuloma than electrocautery.
   - Proximal fascial interposition: Closure of the fascial sheath over the proximal cut end of the vas in a purse-string fashion reduces the risk of re-canalization.
   - Open-ended techniques: The testicular (distal) end of the vas is left open and the proximal end is managed with cautery and fascial

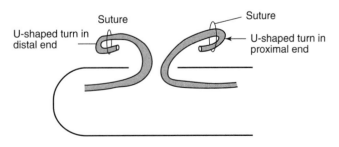

Figure 13.3. Placing the Stitches on the Ends of the Vas.

interposition. This may lead to a decrease in epididymal congestion and thus fewer symptomatic sperm granulomas.

20. Cautery and ligation is our preferred method.
21. Ensure that hemostasis is maintained.
22. The incision is closed with 3/0 synthetic absorbable suture.
23. Repeat the same procedure on the opposite side (Steps 11–22).
24. Patient can go home the same day and resume routine daily activities within 2–3 days.
25. Patients are advised to take painkillers and apply ice packs over a towel or their clothing for no longer than 20 minutes per hour for the first 24 hours. This helps reduce swelling and aids in vasoconstriction.
26. Advise to avoid intercourse for 1 week and to use contraception during intercourse until confirmation of being azoospermic is obtained.
27. Obtain a semen analysis at 12-weeks post-surgery and advise on at least 15 ejaculations in the mean time. If there is sperm then organize another semen anlaysis at 16 weeks.

Procedure: No-Scalpel Technique

1. Steps 1–7, as described in previous section.
2. No-needle jet anesthetic technique involves delivering the anesthetic via an elevated-pressure jet injection instrument, which can be used for this type of vasectomy (Figure 13.4), or alternatively follow Steps 8 and 9 in the previous section.

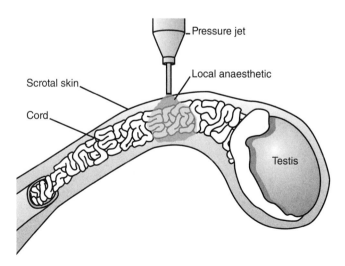

Figure 13.4. No-Needle Jet Anesthetic Technique.

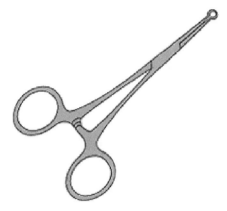

Figure 13.5. Round Vas Clamp.

3. A ringed extracutaneous round vas clamp (Figure 13.5) is used to fixate the vas to the overlying skin between the base of the penis and the top of the testis in the midline raphe. This may be painful if not enough anesthetic is given.
4. Lower the handles of the ringed clamp to elevate the vas.
5. Pierce the skin of the scrotum using a quick, sharp, and single movement using one of the blades of a sharpened dissecting forceps (Figure 13.6) introduced at a 45° angle, in the midline of the vas and downward into the lumen.

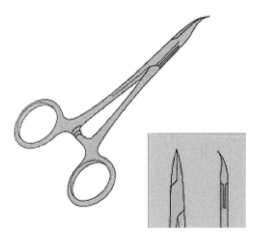

Figure 13.6. Special Dissecting Forceps.

6. Withdraw the blade, close the curved dissecting forceps, and introduce both blades into the same puncture hole at the same angle to a depth of 2–5 mm.
7. The blades of the dissecting forceps are then gently opened to spread the tissue around the vas, and a "back-and-forth" stretching movement is used to create a skin opening twice the diameter of the vas (approximately 4 mm).
8. Introduce the tip of one of the blades of the dissecting forceps into the lumen at a 45° angle and use it to elevate and pull a loop of vas up.
9. Release the ringed forceps, which is grasping the skin at the moment, allowing delivery of the vas deferens with the dissecting forceps.
10. Adjust the ring forceps so that it grasps around the vas. Be careful not to lose the vas into the wound.
11. Puncture the sheath surrounding the vas with one tip of the dissecting forceps and carefully strip the sheath and vasal vessels from the vas, using a longitudinal (not a transverse) motion, with the sharp curved dissecting forceps to yield a bare segment of vas approximately 1.5–2 cm in length. Be careful to avoid blood vessels.
12. Follow Steps 18–22 in the previous section.
13. Repeat these steps for the opposite side using the same midline incision.
14. Follow Steps 24–26 in the previous section.

Complications

Occasional complications include:

- Swelling of the scrotal tissue, bruising, and minor pain
- Sperm granulomas result from leakage of sperm at the testicular end (1–30%)
- Chronic testicular pain (12–52%) secondary to surgical scarring or congestion of the epididymis with dead sperm and fluid requiring removal of the epididymis

Rare complications include:

- Hematoma, which may require evacuation (2%)
- Recanalization, leading to failure of the procedure (0–2%)
- Genitofemoral neuralgia, requiring neurectomy
- Wound infections and epididymitis (1–3 in 500 cases), requiring local wound care and oral antibiotics
- Fistulae: Vasocutaneous; vasovenous; vasourinary; arteriovenous

References

1. Vasoligation. In: *Atlas of Urologic Surgery, 2nd Edition*. Hinman F Jr (Ed). Philadelphia: Saunders; 1998; 362–364.

2. The British Association of Urological Surgeons (Consent forms). http://www.baus.org.uk. Date accessed: May 25, 2007.

3. No-Scalpal Vasectomy. http://www.no-scalpelvasectomy.com. Date accessed: May 25, 2007.

4. Labrecque M, Dufresne C, Barone MA, St-Hilaire K. Vasectomy surgical techniques: a systematic review. BMC Med 2004;2:21.

5. Weiss RS, Li PS. No-needle jet anesthetic technique for no-scalpel vasectomy. J Urol 2005;173(5):1677–1680.

6. Awsare NS, Krishnan J, Boustead GB, Hanbury DC, McNicholas TA. Complications of vasectomy. Ann R Coll Surg Engl 2005;87(6):406–410.

14. Epididymectomy

Hashim Hashim and Paul Abrams

Indications

This is an operation that is seldom indicated and normally used as a last resort, in the treatment of pain. The main indications include post-vasectomy epididymal engorgement, complex epididymal cyst disease, chronic recurrent epididymitis, and epididymal tuberculosis resulting in caseation and a firm expanding mass not responding to antibiotic treatment.

Procedure

1. The most important action, before the operation, is to mark the correct operative side (i.e., right or left) and to include that in the consent form.
2. The operation is normally performed under general/regional anesthesia.
3. Place the patient in the supine position.
4. Shave the scrotum and prepare the lower abdomen, penis, and scrotum with aqueous betadine or chlorhexidine. Drape accordingly.
5. Pull the testis down to relax the cremaster.
6. Grasp the scrotum around and behind the testis with the fingers and thumb of one hand and compress the testis against the anterior scrotal wall to stretch the skin over it (*see* Figure 6.1).
7. One of two incisions can be made (*see* Figure 6.2). They only need to be approximately 3–5 cm long:
   - Unilateral transverse incision, over the testis, within the scrotal folds and between the scrotal vessels. This is the preferred incision if the operation is unilateral.
   - Median raphe incision: allows good access to both testes and results in minimal bleeding with a good post-operative scar.
8. Once the skin is incised, keep the testis under compression and incise the dartos muscle and the underlying cremasteric layers one by one from one edge of the wound to the other. Stop when you reach the tunica vaginalis. Control any bleeding with bipolar diathermy.

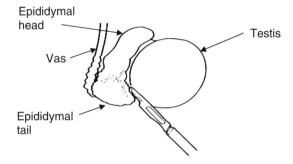

Figure 14.1. Starting Dissection at the Tail of the Epididymis.

9. Push all the scrotal layers away from the testis using a swab. The testis can at this stage be delivered with the tunica vaginalis and then the tunica vaginalis incised. Alternatively, the tunica vaginalis can be opened while the testis is still in the scrotum and then the testis is delivered.

10. Gently pull the testis down to expose the epididymis and cord, and identify the plane between the epididymis and testis.

11. Begin dissection at the tail of the epididymis, keeping close to it to avoid damage to any vessels (Figure 14.1). Starting at the tail allows more epididymis to be dissected before reaching the rete and vessels. However, be careful of the vas at this level.

12. Keep on dissecting until you reach the head of the epididymis. Identify the epididymal branch of the testicular artery and ligate and divide it (Figure 14.2).

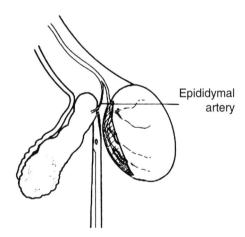

Figure 14.2. Epididymal Artery.

13. The whole epididymis should now be detached from the testis but the vas should still be intact. Clamp, divide, and ligate the vas with 3/0 synthetic absorbable suture.
14. Close the defect in the testis with continuous 3/0 synthetic absorbable suture.
15. The important point is not to damage the arterial supply to the testis. If it does get damaged do not perform an orchidectomy straight away, as there may be collateral supply. If the testis does not appear viable, then an orchidectomy may need to be performed (however ensure that this is included in the consent form).
16. Ensure that hemostasis is maintained before closure.
17. If there is infection or you are worried about bleeding, then a corrugated drain can be inserted coming out through the most dependent part of the scrotum and fixed in place with a 2/0 non-absorbable suture and safety pin (to prevent it from disappearing into the scrotum or falling out).
18. Close the dartos muscle with undyed 3/0 synthetic absorbable suture, in a continuous fashion.
19. Inject 0.5% marcaine into the skin edges and dartos to reduce the post-operative pain.
20. Close the skin with interrupted undyed 4/0 synthetic absorbable suture to avoid staining of the skin. Alternatively, you can use surgical glue or use a 4/0 subcuticular monofilament continuous suture.
21. Cover the wound with non-stick dressing.
22. Give the patient scrotal support to reduce post-operative hematoma.
23. The patient can normally go home the same day and resume routine daily activities within 2–3 days.
24. Patients are advised to take painkillers and apply ice packs over a towel or their clothing for no longer than 20 minutes per hour for the first 24 hours. This helps reduce swelling and aids in vasoconstriction.

Complications

Occasional complications include:

- Infection of the wound, requiring further treatment with antibiotics or surgery
- Bleeding from the wound and formation of scrotal hematoma, requiring surgery
- Potential loss of fertility in the future, even after unilateral procedures

Rare complications include:

- Finding of an unsuspected diagnosis on the histology examination, requiring further treatment
- Patients need to be warned that if the arterial supply to the testis is damaged, then an orchidectomy may need to be performed

References

1. Epididymectomy. In: *Atlas of Urologic Surgery, 2nd Edition*. Hinman F Jr (Ed). Philadelphia: Saunders; 1998; 409–410.
2. The British Association of Urological Surgeons (Consent forms). http://www.baus. org.uk. Date accessed: May 25, 2007.

15. Inguinal Orchidopexy (Orchiopexy)

Hashim Hashim and Paul Abrams

Indications

Orchidopexy is a procedure of securing testis inside the scrotum. It is mainly done in children with cryptorchidism at approximately 6 months of age to minimize the risk of infertility, lower the risk of testicular cancer in undescended testis, lower the risk of traumatic injury to the testicle, prevent the development of an inguinal hernia, prevent testicular torsion in adolescence, and to maintain the appearance of a normal scrotum. Inguinal orchidopexy in children is normally performed by a pediatric surgeon or pediatric urologist. But sometimes, adult urologists with an interest in pediatrics also perform the operation, especially if the testis lies in the superficial inguinal pouch or the inguinal canal (i.e. clinically palpable).

Before the operation, an ultrasound may need to be performed to localize the testis. If it cannot be seen on ultrasound, then a CT – computed tomograph or MRI – magnetic resonance imaging should be performed. If these fail to localize the testis, then laparoscopy is performed with a view to performing a laparoscopic orchidopexy or orchidectomy at the same time.

In adolescents or adult males, orchidopexy is most frequently used in the treatment of testicular torsion and is done through a scrotal approach rather than an inguinal approach (*see* Chapter 6).

We will only describe the procedure for a palpable testis found in the superficial inguinal pouch or in the inguinal canal, under the external oblique aponeurosis, as the other scenarios are more within the remits of a pediatric surgeon or urologist.

Procedure

1. The most important action, before the operation, is to mark the correct operative side (i.e., right or left) and to include that in the consent form.
2. The operation is normally performed under general/regional anesthesia.
3. Place the patient in the supine position, with the legs slightly abducted and feet together.

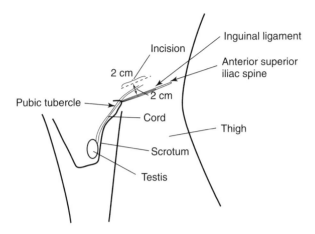

Figure 15.1. Site of Skin Incision.

4. Prepare the lower abdomen, penis, scrotum, and upper thighs with aqueous betadine or chlorhexidine. Drape accordingly.
5. Identify the pubic tubercle and anterior superior iliac spine.
6. Make a 2- to 3-cm incision in the skin, on the appropriate side, just above the superficial inguinal ring and just lateral to the pubic tubercle (Figure 15.1).
7. Incise subcutaneous fat, Camper's fascia, and Scarpa's fascia. Any veins encountered during this step (i.e., the superficial circumflex iliac and superficial inferior epigastric vessels) should be clamped, divided, and ligated with 3/0 synthetic absorbable suture or electrocauterized with diathermy.
8. Be careful when incising Scarpa's fascia, as the testis may be located in the superficial inguinal pouch rather than the inguinal canal. In children, Scarpa's fascia may be confused with the external oblique aponeurosis. Scarpa fascia is smooth, does not have any fibrous bands, has a layer of fat beneath it, and does not glisten like the aponeurosis.
9. Place a self-retaining retractor to open the wound.
10. Identify the external inguinal ring and the fibers of the external oblique. In children the external and internal rings (1–2 cm above the midpoint of the inguinal ligament) are almost superimposed.
11. If the testis is in the superficial inguinal pouch, then it must be freed. Minimal dissection of the cord is required at this level. Compressing the abdomen to increase the intra-abdominal pressure can help the testis to come out of the ring and facilitate dissection.
12. Incise the external oblique fascia laterally along its fibers and extend the incision to the external inguinal ring (Figure 15.2).
13. Free the external oblique from the conjoint tendon and the cremasteric fibers, which would be revealed by this incision.
14. Beware of the ilioinguinal nerve, which lies just beneath the external oblique fascia anterior to the cord. You need to identify and mobilize

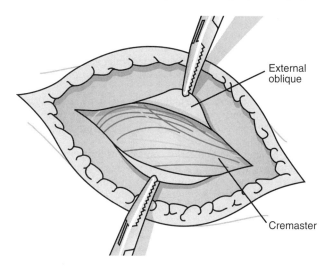

Figure 15.2. Division of the External Oblique Aponeurosis to Reveal the Cremaster.

it so as not to transect it during the procedure, otherwise the patient will get pain and numbness over the skin in the inguinal region, upper part of the thigh, and anterior one-third of scrotum.

15. Divide the internal oblique muscle with scissors or electrocautery and free the space below it with your index finger.

16. Mobilize the testis by dividing the distal gubernacular attachments initially.

17. Identify the testis and put traction on it to make sure that the artery is long enough.

18. Identify the cremasteric muscle fibers and transect them completely to locate the processus (Figure 15.3).

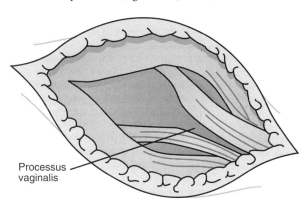

Figure 15.3. Opening the Cremaster Reveals the Porcessus Vaginalis.

19. Open the tunica vaginalis and incise it proximally to the base of the cord.

20. Look for a hernia sac (usually anteromedial to the cord), and retract it medially to reveal the underlying testicular vessels and vas deferens (may be difficult to visualize). Use fine tissue forceps to separate these structures from the hernia sac.

21. Clamp the sac near its edge and mobilize it to the internal ring. There is usually retroperitoneal fat near the internal ring.

22. Separate the cord structures from the peritoneum above the internal inguinal ring.

23. Divide the lateral and posterior connections of the internal spermatic fascia to the tunica to allow medial movement of the testis.

24. Confirm that the sac is empty. It may be worth delaying ligating the sac, as subsequent retraction may tear the closure.

25. Inspect the testis for masses and quality. If poor, perform an orchidectomy (*see* Chapter 8).

26. Gauge the length of the cord by pulling the testis over the symphysis. If more cord is required, then dissect more tunica and cremasteric fibers from the cord around the internal ring. You may need to continue dissection retroperitoneally.

27. If further cord length is needed, the Prentiss maneuver can be used. Locate and clamp, divide, and ligate the inferior epigastric artery and vein separately (or pass the testis under them). Open the transversalis fascia and the internal inguinal ring by dividing the internal oblique muscles and more of the lateral spermatic fascia. The inguinal incision also may be lengthened to enable this dissection.

28. Continue dissection of the cord, using peanut dissectors, in the retroperitoneal space, upward in the direction of the lower pole of the kidney.

29. At this stage if the hernia sac is empty, twist the sac and transfix it near the internal inguinal ring by holding it vertically using the clamp and placing a 2/0 synthetic absorbable suture through the sac. Tie the ends of the stitch into a half hitch and then completely encircle the neck of the sac and tie the suture.

30. Pass the index finger, clamp, or balloon catheter (*see* Chapter 9) along the usual course of testicular descent into the scrotum until it reaches a natural position (Figure 15.4).

31. Make 2-cm transverse incision through the scrotal skin over the finger or clamp. Do not incise the dartos (Figure 15.4).

32. Free the skin from the dartos using blunt dissection with a mosquito clamp to develop a 2-cm–deep subdartos pouch.

33. Make a small incision in the dartos, which is stretched over the finger, and place an Allis clamp on both edges.

34. Insert a tissue clamp through the incision in the scrotum and dartos up towards the inguinal wound by following the finger or clamp already in the scrotum.

35. Clamp the edges of the tunica albuginea and draw the testis down into the scrotum through the scrotal opening and into the punch between the dartos and skin. Make sure you do not rotate the cord (Figures 15.5 and 15.6).

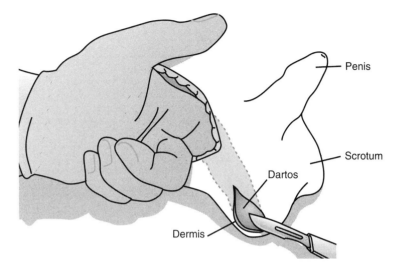

Figure 15.4. Making a Tract for the Testis and Incising the Skin Transversely.

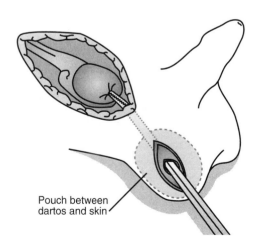

Figure 15.5. Grabbing the Tunica Albuginea and Bringing the Testis Down.

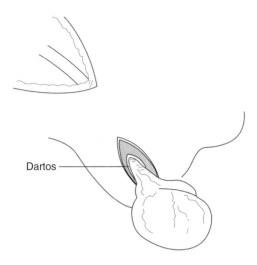

Figure 15.6. Bringing Testis Out Through Dartos and Scrotal Incision.

36. Different methods of testicular fixation are available and each has its advantagaes and disadvantages:
    - Subcutaneous pouch with suture fixation (suture the upper lateral or medial pole with the skin) or a sutureless subdartos pouch (causes least fibrosis, but can twist)
    - Absorbable (cause more fibrosis) versus permanent sutures (sutures can be felt through the skin)
    - Tunica vaginalis fixation (less secure) versus tunica albuginea fixation (can cause testicular parenchymal damage)
37. Close the scrotal skin with interrupted undyed 4/0 synthetic absorbable sutures (can include the tunica albuginea with one of the stitches; see above).
38. Close the inguinal wound. Approximate the transversalis fascia over the cord with interrupted 3/0 synthetic absorbable sutures.
39. The internal oblique muscle can either be approximated or sutured to the shelving edge of the inguinal ligament with interrupted 3/0 synthetic absorbable sutures.
40. Close the external oblique muscle aponeurosis with interrupted 3/0 absorbable sutures to create a new external ring, but do not make it too tight.
41. Appose Scarpa's fascia in an interrupted fashion using 4/0 synthetic absorbable suture.
42. Inject 0.5% marcaine into the skin edges and fascia and along the ilioinguinal nerve to reduce the post-operative pain as well as into the scrotal incision.

43. Close the skin with subcuticular 4/0 monofilament absorbable continuous suture. Alternatively, you can use surgical glue.
44. Cover both wounds with a dressing of your choice and give the patient a scrotal support.
45. The patient can normally go home the same day with oral analgesia. Advise patient to keep the surgical area dry for 3 days.
46. Follow up the patient in 1 month and in 6–12 months post-operatively to check the testis location, size, and viability.
47. It may be worth doing a semen analysis in children when they reach the age of 18 years.

Complications

Occasional complications include:

- Bruising or bleeding, which resolves slowly but may require surgical evacuation
- Failure of the testicle to remain in the scrotum
- Inadequate testis position (10% of patients) owing to incomplete retroperitoneal dissection, which may need a second surgical procedure to bring the testis down to the ideal position
- Testicular atrophy (5% of cases) owing to devascularization during dissection of the cord
- Accidental division of the vas deferens (1–2% of patients), which may require a further surgical procedure to repair it

Rare complications include:

- Damage to the blood vessels and other structures in the spermatic cord, leading to eventual loss of the testicle
- Infection of incision or scrotal contents, requiring further treatment with antibiotics
- Recurrence of hernia can occur, needing further treatment
- Development of a hydrocele, requiring further surgical intervention
- Later development of testicular cancer, necessitating orchiectomy and insertion of prosthesis
- Potential loss of fertility in the future

References

1. Inguinal orchiopexy. In: *Atlas of Urologic Surgery, 2nd Edition*. Hinman F Jr (Ed). Philadelphia: Saunders; 1998; 308–315.
2. The British Association of Urological Surgeons (Consent forms). http://www.baus.org.uk. Date accessed: May 25, 2007.

16. Varicocelectomy

Hashim Hashim and Paul Abrams

Indications

Varicocelectomy is the most commonly performed operation for the treatment of male infertility. Treatment is either by radiological embolization or surgery. Indications for intervention include a varicocele associated with infertility, painful varicoceles, and a large varicocele in a child or adolescent with testicular atrophy or recurrent varicocele after previous embolization or surgery. There are three common surgical approaches: subinguinal (Marmar), inguinal (Ivanissevich), and abdominal (Palomo).

The sub-inguinal will not be discussed, as it is a significantly more difficult procedure than the inguinal approach and probably should be reserved for surgeons who perform the operation frequently. Also, at this level more veins are encountered surrounding the artery. Furthermore, the testicular artery divides into two or three branches, making arterial identification and preservation more difficult.

Procedure: Inguinal Varicocelectomy

1. The most important action, before the operation, is to mark the correct operative side (i.e., right or left) and to include that in the consent form.
2. The operation is normally performed under general/regional anesthesia, but can be performed under local anesthesia.
3. Place the patient in the supine position.
4. Shave the scrotum and lower abdomen and prepare the lower abdomen, penis, and scrotum with aqueous betadine or chlorhexidine. Drape accordingly.
5. Locate the external inguinal ring by invaginating the scrotal skin up into the inguinal region.
6. Make an inguinal incision in the skin, on the appropriate side, beginning at the external inguinal ring and extending 3–4 cm laterally parallel to the inguinal ligament or along Langer's skin lines (Figure 16.1).
7. Incise subcutaneous fat, Camper's fascia, and Scarpa's fascia. Any veins encountered during this step should be clamped, divided, and

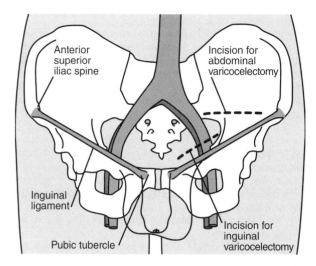

Figure 16.1. Inguinal and Abdominal Varicocelectomy Incisions.

ligated with 3/0 synthetic absorbable suture or electrocauterized with diathermy.

8. Place a self-retaining retractor to open the wound.
9. Identify the external inguinal ring and the fibers of the external oblique. Incise the external oblique (the length of the skin incision) along its fibers, starting from the external ring.
10. Beware of the ilioinguinal nerve, which lies just beneath the external oblique fascia. You need to identify and mobilize it so as not to resect it during the procedure.
11. Grasp both edges of the external oblique with clamps. Alternatively, placing a 3/0 absorbable suture at the lateral end of the external oblique incision facilitates later closure.
12. Bluntly dissect the spermatic cord to expose the pubic tubercle. This can be done with peanut dissectors and by sweeping the index finger gently along the pubic tubercle so that the index finger can be placed under and around the cord.
13. Place a ring clamp or a Penrose drain around the cord to secure it as you would for an inguinal orchidectomy (*see* Chapter 8).
14. Pull the testis out of the scrotum by pulling the cord near the pubic tubercle and also applying upward pressure on the scrotum under the testis. Delivering the testis allows visualization of all the veins draining the testis, especially most of the external spermatic, scrotal, or guber-nacular collaterals.
15. Clamp, divide, and ligate all the external spermatic, scrotal, or guber-nacular collaterals.

16. Return the testis to its normal position.
17. Now open the external and internal spermatic fascia of the cord to expose the varicoceles. Some surgeons suggest using magnifying loupes for this part of the procedure, as they provide more magnification of the small testicular artery and lymphatics.
18. Irrigate with 1% papaverine solution to dilate the artery and help visualize the testicular artery (0.5- to 1.5-mm diameter) pulsations. Alternatively, you can use a 3-mm high-frequency (24 MHz) Doppler probe to identify the artery.
19. Dissect the artery to free it of all surrounding tissues, including veins and lymphatics. The artery is usually on the under-surface of a large vein or it may have two large veins, one on either side.
20. Place a vessel loop around the artery to allow easy identification.
21. If it is difficult to identify the artery, dissect the cord carefully beginning with the largest veins.
22. Strip the veins of any adherent lymphatics. The artery may then become apparent.
23. Clamp, ligate, and divide all the veins in succession within the cord with 4/0 synthetic non-absorbable sutures. You can use electrocautery for veins smaller than 0.5 mm.
24. Do not ligate the vasal (veins along the vas) veins, as they provide venous return, unless they are greater than 3 mm in diameter. The vas deferens is always accompanied by two sets of vessels and at least one set needs to be preserved.
25. Inspect and feel the cord to verify that all veins have been identified and ligated.
26. At the end of the procedure you should be left with the testicular artery, lymphatics, and vas deferens with its vessels.
27. Remove the clamp and ensure that the cord returns to its normal position.
28. Ensure hemostasis.
29. Close the external oblique fascia in continuous running fashion using 3/0 synthetic absorbable suture.
30. Appose Scarpa's fascia in an interrupted fashion using 3/0 synthetic absorbable suture.
31. Approximate Camper's fascia in an interrupted fashion using 4/0 synthetic absorbable suture.
32. Inject 0.5% marcaine into the skin edges and fascia and along the ilioinguinal nerve to reduce the post-operative pain.
33. Close the skin with subcuticular 3/0 monofilament absorbable continuous suture. Alternatively, you can use surgical glue or skin clips (need to be removed in 10 days post-operatively).
34. Cover the wound with a dressing of your choice.
35. Give the patient a scrotal support to reduce post-operative hematoma.
36. The patient can normally go home the same day with analgesia and resume routine activities in 2–3 days.

37. Advantages of this approach include:
    - Easier in patients who are obese
    - Requires less assistance
    - Can be readily done under local anesthesia
    - Allows spermatic cord structures to be pulled out of wound and identified, and provides easy access to the testis

Procedure: Abdominal Varicocelectomy

1. The most important action, before the operation, is to mark the correct operative side (i.e., right or left) and to include that in the consent form.
2. The operation is normally performed under general/regional anesthesia, but can be performed under local anesthesia.
3. Place the patient in the supine position with the head elevated approximately 10° (reverse Trendelenburg). This allows filling of the veins.
4. Shave lower abdomen and prepare the lower abdomen, penis, and scrotum with aqueous betadine or chlorhexidine. Drape accordingly.
5. Make a 4- to 5-cm skin incision along Langer's line, two fingerbreadths medial to the anterior superior iliac spine over the internal inguinal ring and lateral to the line of the femoral artery (Figure 16.1).
6. Incise the subcutaneous fat until you reach the external oblique aponeurosis.
7. Incise the external oblique aponeurosis along its fibers. Be careful of the ilioinguinal nerve, which lies directly beneath it.
8. Separate the internal oblique muscle fibers bluntly using retractors. This will reveal the transversus abdominis muscle.
9. Incise the transversus abdominis muscle and enter the retroperitoneal space 3–5 cm above the inguinal ligament.
10. Place a self-retaining retractor in the wound and push the peritoneum medially. This should reveal testicular artery and vein retroperitoneally, near the ureter, femoral artery, and inferior epigastric artery and vein, as they rise to join the vas. Pulling on the ipsilateral testis can help identify the cord structures.
11. Pass a vessel loop behind the vessels and elevate them.
12. Drip 1% papaverine over the vessels to dilate the artery and make it visibly pulsatile.
13. Seperate the veins from the artery and lymphatics. Ligating the testicular artery at this level is not very harmful, as there is usually a collateral circulation to the testis from the cremasteric and vasal vessels.
14. Clamp, divide, and ligate the dilated veins. There are usually two of them (Figure 16.2).
15. Ensure hemostasis and close the layers one by one.

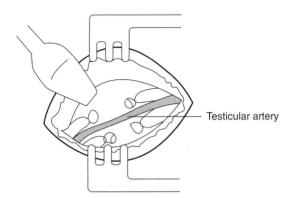

Figure 16.2. Two Testicular Veins Divided to Reveal the Testicular Artery In Abdominal Varicocelectomy.

16. Close the transverses abdominus in a continuous running fashion using 3/0 synthetic absorbable suture.
17. Approximate the internal oblique muscle in an interrupted fashion using 3/0 synthetic absorbable suture.
18. Close the external oblique in an interrupted fashion using 4/0 synthetic absorbable suture.
19. Close the skin with subcuticular 3/0 monofilament absorbable continuous suture. Alternatively, you can use surgical glue or skin clips (need to be removed in 10 days post-operatively).
20. Cover the wound with a dressing of your choice.
21. The patient can normally go home the same day with analgesia and resume routine activities in 2–3 days.
22. Advantages of this technique include:
    • Isolating the testicular veins proximally, closer to the point of drainage into the left renal vein. Thus only one or two large veins are present, requiring fewer ligations.
    • The testicular artery has not yet branched, and is often distinctly separate from the internal spermatic veins.

Complications

Occasional complications include:

• Hydrocele formation caused by lymphatic obstruction (3–33%, with an average incidence of approximately 7%)

- Testicular artery injury, resulting in testicular atrophy and/or impaired spermatogenesis leading to loss of future fertility
- Varicocele recurrence (0.6–45%). Higher in the abdominal approach, because parallel inguinal or retroperitoneal collaterals may bypass the ligated retroperitoneal veins and rejoin the internal spermatic (testicular) vein proximal to the site of ligation and the dilated cremasteric veins cannot be identified.

Rare complications include

- Bleeding, resulting in a hematoma or retroperitoneal bleeding may require further surgery to stop the bleeding
- Injury to the ilioinguinal nerve, resulting in loss of sensation to the ipsilateral groin and lateral hemiscrotum
- Infection of incision, requiring further treatment with antibiotics

References

1. Varicocele ligation. In: *Atlas of Urologic Surgery, 2nd Edition*. Hinman F Jr (Ed). Philadelphia: Saunders; 1998; 352–358.
2. Goldstein M. Chapter 44: Surgical management of male infertility and other scrotal disorders. *In: Campbell's Urology, 8th Edition*. Walsh PC, Retik AB, Vaughan ED Jr, Wein AJ (Eds). Philadelphia: Saunders; 2002.

17. Circumcision

Christopher Wolter and Roger Dmochowski

Indications

Circumcision is the term for a number of technical procedures to remove the penile foreskin, or prepuce. In adults, there are a number of medical indications for this procedure. The most common indication is phimosis, a tightness or constriction of the prepuce over the glans, making it difficult to retract. The converse of this is paraphimosis, in which a retracted foreskin is unable to be replaced, usually resulting in pain and edema of the glans. This is considered a relative emergency, and surgical reduction may be necessary if the foreskin is unable to be reduced manually. Preputial tumors or lesions, recurrent balanitis and/or balanoposthitis, pain, discomfort and redundancy round out the more common medical indications for circumcision (1). Patients may also elect to undergo this procedure for cosmetic or personal reasons.

In children, there is ongoing controversy over the reasons for circumcision. Although the majority of circumcisions in boys are done in the neonatal period for religious, cultural, and personal reasons, there are some medical arguments for circumcision in this patient population. Circumcision in male infants has shown to decrease rates of urinary tract infection by close to 20-fold. In addition to this, there is a reduced transmission of some sexually transmitted diseases, including HIV. It is also believed to decrease transmission of human papilloma virus, thus reducing cervical cancer risk. A longstanding argument for circumcision has also been that it reduces the incidence of penile cancer to almost zero, though the same result can be had from adequate hygiene in patients without circumcision.

Procedure

Adults

1. Place the patient on the table in the supine position. Shave and prep the skin with an appropriate antiseptic solution, and drape the genitals.
2. This procedure can be done under either general or local anesthesia. If local is chosen, it is important to use a local anesthetic without epi-

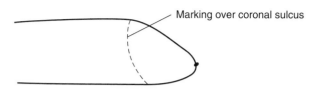

Figure 17.1. Marking the Proximal Incision.

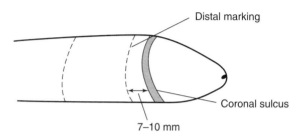

Figure 17.2. Marking the Distal Incision After Retracting the Foreskin.

nephrine. A dorsal penile nerve block should be placed along with a ring block of the penis *(2)* *(see* Section 1).

3. With the foreskin in its normal position and the penis slightly on stretch or the suprapubic fat pad depressed *(1)*, the coronal sulcus is first marked with a marking pen for the proximal incision (Figure 17.1). The foreskin is then reduced, and the distal incision is marked usually 7–10 mm from the coronal ridge (Figure 17.2). This mark should include the frenulum.

4. With a scalpel, make the proximal incision through the skin and down to Buck's fascia. Repeat with the distal incision. Take care when going through the ventral surface near the frenulum. The frenulum should pull apart and distally after being incised.

5. With only the dartos holding the foreskin on, there are many ways to completely remove the foreskin. Here we will describe two techniques:

   • Sleeve technique (Figure 17.3): Use hemostats to place traction dorsally initially and dissect the foreskin from the underlying Buck's

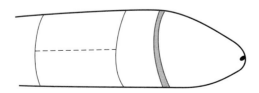

Figure 17.3. The Sleeve Technique – Joining the Two Incisions Together.

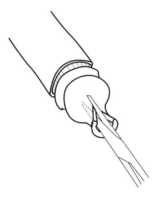

Figure 17.4. Dorsal Slit to Join the Two Incisions Together.

fascia with either sharp dissection or electrocautery. Ensure the glans is protected. Completely excise all attachments.
- Dorsal Slit: Reduce the foreskin and, while protecting the glans, incise the foreskin dorsally to join the two incisions (Figure 17.4). Grasp the edges with hemostats and use electrocautery to dissect the remaining dartos attachments to free the foreskin *(3)*.
6. Carefully obtain hemostasis using fine vascular forceps and electro-cautery. Do not over-cauterize the skin edges.
7. Using a 3/0 synthetic absorbable suture, first place a U-stitch at the ventral midline. This should reapproxmate both the median raphe and the frenulum. Leave the stitch long and tag with a hemostat to aid in traction.
8. Place simple interrupted 3/0 synthetic absorbable sutures in the remaining quadrants and tag these with hemostats as well. This will aid the solo surgeon in traction and positioning.
9. Complete the skin closure with an appropriate number of interrupted sutures to close the remaining gaps in the anastomosis (Figure 17.5).

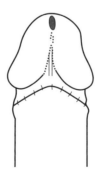

Figure 17.5. The Final Outcome of the Two Ends Joined Together.

10. The frenulum may require additional horizontal sutures.
11. The suture line may be covered with antibiotic ointment or petroleum gauze, and then a sterile dressing is applied. The penis can then be gently wrapped, with great care being taken to not place the dressing too tightly. This can result in necrosis distally if wrapped too tight.
12. The patient can go home the same day. The dressing can be removed in 24–48 hours. He should be instructed avoid sexual activity of any kind for 4–6 weeks until the sutures dissolve. A short course of analgesics may be necessary and should be provided.
13. If non-absorbable sutures are used then these will need to be removed in 10–14 days.

Complications

Potential complications most commonly seen *(1)*:

- Bleeding, requiring intervention ranging from manual pressure to surgical exploration
- Infection, requiring antibiotics and/or surgical intervention
- Pain, either during the procedure from inadequate anesthesia, or postoperatively
- Poor cosmesis
- Incomplete removal of foreskin
- Removal of too much foreskin, resulting in penile angulation, shortening, or discomfort
- Breakdown or disruption of the suture line caused by premature sexual activity or erection
- Altered sensation with intercourse
- Persistence if absorbable stitches after 3/4 weeks requiring removal.

References

1. Holman JR, Stuessi KA. Adult circumcision. Am Fam Physician 1999;59(6): 1514–1518.
2. Wakefield SE, Elewa AA. Adult circumcision under local anaesthetic. Br J Urol 1995;75:96.
3. Circumcision. In: *Atlas of Urologic Surgery, 2nd Edition.* Hinman F Jr (Ed). Philadelphia: Saunders; 1998; 167–173.
4. The British Association of Urological Surgeons (Consent forms). http://www.baus. org.uk. Date accessed: May 25, 2007.

18. Optical Urethrotomy

Christopher Wolter and Roger Dmochowski

Indications

Optical urethrotomy is a procedure in which a urethral stricture is incised under direct visualization endoscopically. A specialized scope called an urethrotome (Figure 18.1) is used. This instrument has a knife blade that is deployed by the surgeon, and which faces in the upward direction (1). In general, it is indicated for first time strictures as long as they are relatively short in length, and do not appear overly dense by cystoscopy. It can be utilized for recurrent small strictures after urethroplasty as well. More complex urethral strictures can be incised as well with this technique, although the failure rate is generally much higher. Patients who would otherwise not tolerate a more extensive open reconstruction are also candidates.

Procedure

1. Preoperative consent should be obtained. The patient should have an understanding that recurrence is possible. Pre-operative imaging to confirm stricture location and length is necessary, as well as to assess for multiple strictures.
2. This procedure is usually done under general anesthesia, but can be done under local in select patients using intra-urethral lidocaine jelly.
3. Pre-operative antibiotics should be given.
4. Place the patient on a cystoscopy table in the dorsal lithotomy position. It is not necessary to have the patient in an exaggerated position.
5. Set up the operative field as is done for rigid cystoscopy (*see* Chapter 24). This should include standard skin preparation and draping.
6. Using the optical urethrotome, enter the urethral meatus with the scope. A 0° lens should be used. It is important that you have the correct working elements, and make sure you are familiar with them. The optical urethrotome works by movement of the thumb as opposed to the resectoscope, which works by movement of the fingers.

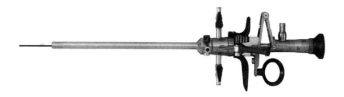

Figure 18.1. Optical Urethrotome (Olympus) With Blade (0° Endoscope Needs to Be Used).

7. Continue urethroscopy until the strictured area is encountered. Pass a ureteral catheter or guidewire through the lumen of the stricture if possible. This will aid in guiding where to incise the stricture *(2)*.
8. After passing the guidewire or catheter, leave this in the urethra and remove the scope. Reinsert the scope alongside the guidewire.
9. Deploy the cutting blade (corrugated, straight, or semi-circular) of the urethrotome and incise the stricture at the 12 o'clock position. This is accomplished by inserting the blade into the lumen of the stricture and withdrawing it, while placing slight traction in the upward direction while withdrawing the entire scope *(3)*. This should be done in a very carefully controlled manner so as to avoid sudden deep cuts or too long of an incision.
10. Reassess the stricture. If it appears to be open, attempt to advance the scope through the incised area. If it advances easily, no further incision is necessary. If the strictured area is still not open, or the scope does not advance, repeat the previous step. For more dense or narrow strictures, it may be necessary to incise in multiple areas.
11. Once the stricture is opened, advance the scope completely into the bladder and drain the bladder of urine. Then fill the bladder with irrigating fluid.
12. Leaving the guidewire in place, carefully visualize the urethra and strictured area while withdrawing the scope. Biopsy any areas of the urethra or stricture that look clinically suspicious.
13. Over the guidewire, place a 16- to 20-F Council-tip catheter (*see* Chapter 19) and advance it into the bladder. Confirm that irrigant flows back from the catheter and withdraw the guidewire. Inflate the balloon.
14. The catheter should remain for a short term (2–5 days).
15. After removal, the patient can be started on a course of intermittent self-catheterization *(3)*. A 16- to 18-F hydrophilic catheter should be employed. Frequency of catheterization can vary from daily to twice weekly, depending on the severity of the initial stricture and clinical suspicion of the risk of recurrence.

Complications

- Recurrence of the stricture. Any degree of recurrence can be found, and the strictured area can be worse than previously encountered, and can manifest as complete retention.
- Pain, either during the procedure if done under local anesthesia, or after the procedure. This can include pain with catheterization or dysuria.
- Infection, including cystitis, requiring antibiotics
- Periurethral abscess, requiring drainage
- Urethral fistula, requiring prolonged catheterization or surgical repair
- Bleeding, which may require catheterization to tamponade the urethra

References

1. Smith PJB, Dunn M, Dounis A. The early results of treatment of stricture of the male urethra using the Sachse optical urethrotome. Br J Urol 1979;51:224–228.
2. Disorders of the penis and male urethra. In: *Smith's General Urology, 16th Edition*. Tanagho EA, McAninch JW (Eds). McGraw-Hill; 2003; 612–626.
3. Lawrence WT, MacDonagh RP. Treatment of urethral stricture disease by internal urethrotomy followed by intermittent "low friction" self catheterization: preliminary communication. J R Soc Med 1988;81(3):136–139.

19. Urethral Dilation

Christopher Wolter and Roger Dmochowski

Indications

Urethral dilation is a procedure by which the urethral diameter is expanded by passage of sequentially larger sounds or dilators. Today, its main indication is for male stricture disease and is typically reserved for the setting of catheter placement or to allow for cystoscopy. It should not be used as definitive treatment of male stricture disease, as it will typically return after dilation alone. This is better suited to optical urethrotomy or urethroplasty. In addition it is no longer routinely recommended for women. Regardless of how it is done, the patient usually requires a period of catheterization afterwards. Here, the procedure discussed will entail dilation over a guidewire. Although dilation with filiforms and followers has historically been used, we do not recommend it unless the stricture is definitely confined to the penile urethra or fossa navicularis.

Procedure

1. Obtain consent for the procedure. The patient should expect to be catheterized for several days afterwards.
2. Often the procedure needs to be done in the setting of urinary retention. Manipulation of the urethra and the tissue trauma can cause bacteremia. Cover the patient with antibiotics.
3. This can be done under local anesthesia, or general if the patient will not tolerate it awake. If done under local, parenteral analgesia is helpful, as is intra-urethral lidocaine jelly.
4. Set up the patient for cystourethroscopy. If performing at the bedside under local anesthesia, flexible cystoscopy is used. If performing under general anesthesia in the operating room, prepare for rigid cystoscopy.
5. Proceed with cystourethroscopy. Advance into the urethra until the strictured area is encountered.
6. Through the working channel of the scope, pass a flexible tipped guidewire (Figure 19.1) through the stricture. Be careful to pass the wire through the true lumen of the stricture. Do not raise a false passage. Advance carefully, and there should be little to no resistance. If resistance is encountered early, withdraw the wire and try again.

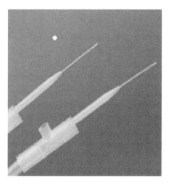

Figure 19.1. Flexible-Tip Guidewire (Bard).

When performing the procedure on a patient who is awake, they should be able to tell you when the wire is in their bladder, as this causes distinct irritation to them.

7. If, after several unsuccessful attempts at passing the guidewire, you are not able to gain access into the bladder, consider stopping and proceeding with suprabubic catheterization (*see* Chapter 25). This should be a rare occurrence.

8. When the wire is in the bladder, you may proceed with dilation.

9. Start dilation by sequentially introducing Heyman dilators (filiforms [Figure 19.2], followers [Figure 19.3], and Goodwin sounds [Figure 19.4]) over the guidewire. Start with the 12-F size. Use plenty of lubrication on the dilator and provide slight counter-traction on guidewire, taking care not to pull it out. Resistance will be encountered at the site of the strictured area. Advance the dilator all the way into the bladder. There should be a trickle of urine from the dilator when it is in the bladder.

10. Proceed with the next size dilator (usually 14 F). Pass in a similar manner. Continue to sequentially dilate until 20–22 F. Generally speak-

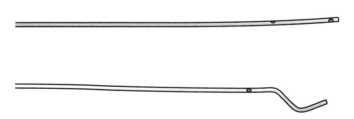

Figure 19.2. Heyman Filiform Catheters: Straight-Tip and Coude-Tip (Bard). Manufactured From Radiopaque Polyurethane With a Stainless Steel Wire Stylet.

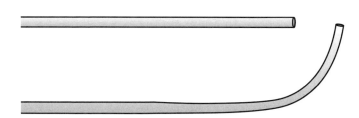

Figure 19.3. Heyman Followers: Straight-Tip and Coude-Tip (Bard). Made of a Special-Formula Pliable Plastic.

ing, you want to dilate to 1–2 sizes greater than the catheter you intend to pass (e.g., dilate to 20 F to pass a 16- or 18-F catheter).

11. If you are not planning on passing the catheter immediately and want to perform cystoscopy, do so now along side the guidewire.

12. When ready, pass a well-lubricated Council-tipped catheter (Figure 19.5) over the guidewire and advance it into the bladder. The rubber catheter lacks the stiffness of the dilator, so firm traction on the wire is necessary. It is easy to pull the wire out, be careful not to do this until you have return of urine through the catheter.

13. If you do not have access to a Council-tipped catheter, you can use a regular two-way Foley and cut, using scissors, the tip of it. Inflate the balloon first and then cut only a small part of the tip of the catheter to allow the guidewire through. It is important that you inflate the balloon so that when you cut the tip you can see if the balloon deflates instantaneously, which means you have cut a large piece and will need to use another catheter. Once the cut is made, deflate the balloon and insert over the guidewire.

14. Once the catheter is in the bladder, remove the wire completely and inflate the balloon.

15. Depending on how dense the stricture is, you will need to vary how long the catheter is left in. The patient should expect to have it from 3–7 days typically, though it can be left in longer if clinically warranted.

16. After the catheter is in for a sufficient time, a voiding trial can be attempted. If successful, the patient should understand that the stric-

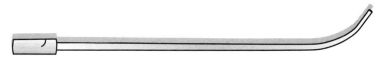

Figure 19.4. Goodwin Sound (Bard): Complements the Heyman System.

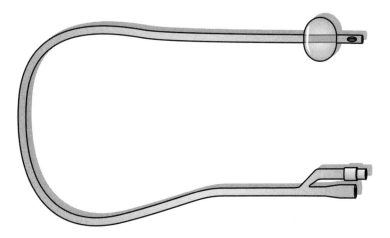

Figure 19.5. Council (Open)-Tip Catheter (Bard).

ture can recur, and a more definitive procedure may need to be undertaken in the future.

17. Patient can be advised to perform intermittent self-catheterization to try to prevent the structure from recurring.

Complications

- Bleeding, usually self-limited and tamponaded by the catheter
- Infection, requiring antibiotics
- Creation of a false passage in the urethra
- Inability to complete the procedure, requiring conversion to suprapubic catheterization
- Pain or discomfort during the procedure
- Recurrence of the stricture

Reference

1. The British Associate of Urological Surgeons (Consent forms). http://www.baus.org. uk. Date accessed: May 25, 2007.

20. Injectables

Christopher Wolter, Roger Dmochowski, and Hashim Hashim

Indications

Injectable therapy for stress urinary incontinence is a well-tolerated, efficacious, minimally invasive treatment. There are several injectable agents available on the market today. Collagen is the agent most written about and has the longest follow-up available, but the newer agents, including carbon-coated zirconium beads, ethylene vinyl alcohol, and calcium hydroxylapatite, all seem to show similar efficacy. Each product varies slightly in its viscosity and injectable carrier gel. The agents themselves serve as a bulking substance for the urethra, which increases outlet resistance. Injectable agents are indicated in conditions of stress incontinence and, more specifically, in conditions of intrinsic sphincteric deficiency. In males, they can be used for post-prostatectomy incontinence as well. We recommend a urodynamic workup in all patients before proceeding.

Procedure

In Females (1)

1. Obtain consent for the procedure. Be sure to inform the patient that there is a risk for urinary retention and that they may need to perform self-catheterization. They should also be aware that more than one injection is likely necessary.
2. Check a urine culture before the procedure, as well as a urinalysis the day of the procedure. Do not proceed if there is bacteriuria.
3. The procedure can usually be accomplished with local anesthesia.
4. Set up the patient for a typical rigid cystoscopy (*see* Chapter 24), prepping the vagina and perineum with aqueous betadine or chlorhexidine. The scope used will be a 21-F rigid cystoscope with a working channel. A long needle for the injectable agent will also need to be set up.
5. Place lidocaine jelly in the urethra and over the meatus and leave on for several minutes.
6. Begin cystoscopy as you normally would, empty the bladder. Have the needle advanced through the working channel of the scope to have it ready. A syringe with 1% plain lidocaine should be connected first.

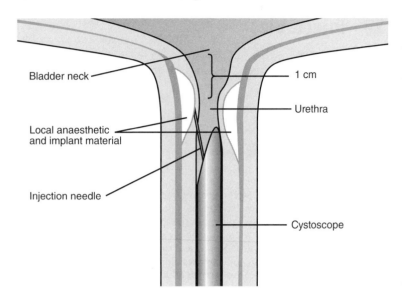

Figure 20.1. Anatomy and Injection of Local Anesthetic at 3 and 9 O'clock Position and Implant Material.

7. Withdraw the cystoscope to approximately 1 cm distal to the bladder neck. Advance your needle through the scope (Figure 20.1). Insert the needle in the submucosa at the 3-, 6-, or 9-o'clock position. Inject 1 cc of lidocaine. This should raise a nice wheal, dissecting the submucosal space. Give the patient time for the initial sting from this to subside.

8. Without withdrawing the needle, remove the lidocaine syringe from the needle and replace it with the syringe containing the injectable bulking agent.

9. In the same space the lidocaine was injected, now inject the bulking agent. There should be good coaptation of the urethra seen as the material is injected. Do not over-inject and rupture the mucosa. Leave the bladder full and withdraw the scope and needle.

10. Alternatively, you can inject the local anesthesia and the agent at the 3- and 9-o'clock positions (Figure 20.1).

11. Have the patient attempt to void before she leaves. If unable to do so, teach her clean intermittent catheterization.

12. The patient should be reassessed in 4 weeks. If there is still some degree of incontinence, the procedure can be repeated.

In Males (2)

1. Obtain consent for the procedure as you would for women. In addition, the pre-procedure work-up includes urinalysis and culture.
2. The set and equipment is also the same as in the previous steps.
3. For males, this procedure is usually effective under local anesthesia, but may be less well tolerated than in females. Consider doing the procedure in the operating room in case general anesthesia needs to be used. The use of intra-urethral lidocaine is very helpful in any case.
4. Proceed with rigid cystoscopy as you normally would in a male.
5. Enter the bladder, drain it, and with the irrigant running, withdraw the scope and identify the area of the external sphincter.
6. Just proximal to the sphincter, insert the needle in the submucosal space and inject the agent on either side of the urethra. Coaptation should be seen after the agent is injected.
7. Leaving he bladder full, remove the scope. Have the patient try to void after the procedure. If they are unable to do so or have difficulty, teach them clean intermittent catheterization.
8. The follow-up is the same as for women in the previous steps.

Zuidex Procedure in Females

This is a procedure that can be performed on an outpatient basis in the examination room in approximately 20 minutes with local anesthesia. It uses a gel that is a copolymer of stabilized non-animal hyaluronic acid and dextranomer (3). It uses four syringes held by an IMPLACER to inject the gel. The same precautions apply as before.

1. Prepare the patient as for a regular flexible cystoscopy (see Chapter 23), including the local anesthetic jelly.
2. Perform a vaginal examination and assess the length of the urethra with your index finger.
3. Assemble the equipment as is described in the manufacturers leaflet.
4. Introduce IMPLACER (with the tube covering the needles) so that the top of the tube is located approximately at the mid-urethra level (Figure 20.2). It is important that the tube does not move backwards during the insertion into the urethra. To avoid this, apply pressure on the thumb grip of the tube while inserting.
5. Pull back the tube to release the needles within the urethra. The needle tips are then located approximately at the mid-urethra level (Figure 20.3).

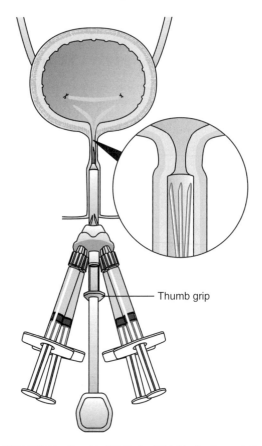

Thumb grip

Figure 20.2. IMPLACER Tube Placed in Mid-Urethra With Needles Covered, Close to Urethral Sphincter Muscle.

6. Push the first syringe to its bottom position in order to penetrate the mucosa. Inject the contents of the syringe into the submucosa (Figure 20.4). Leave the emptied syringe in place. Going clockwise, repeat this maneuver with the remaining three syringes.

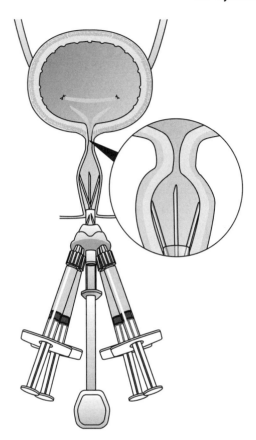

Figure 20.3. Needles Released in Mid-Urethra by Pulling Back the Implacer Tube to Expose the Needles, Which Are Then Pushed Forward to Penetrate the Mucosa.

7. Remove the syringes with the needles one by one and thereafter IMPLACER. The syringes, needles, and IMPLACER must be discarded after the treatment session.
8. Post-procedure precautions apply as before.

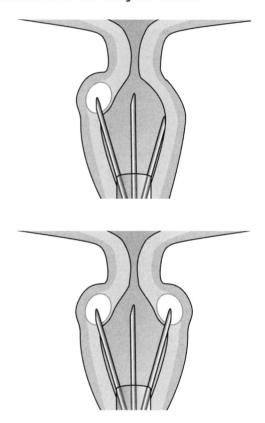

Figure 20.4. Bevels of the Needles Positioned Outwards to Allow More Accurate Placement of Gel in the Submucosal Plane.

Complications

- Bleeding
- Urinary tract infection, or worse, infection of the injection site
- Urinary retention
- Recurrence of incontinence, requiring additional injections after initial efficacy
- Urinary urgency and frequency, possibly requiring medical therapy

References

1. O'Connell HE, McGuire EJ, Aboseif S, Usui A. Transurethral collagen therapy in women. J Urol 1995;154(4):1463–1465.
2. Aboseif SR, O'Connell HE, Usui A, McGuire EJ. Collagen injection for intrinsic sphincteric deficiency in men. J Urol 1996;155(1):10–13.
3. Zuidex International. http://www.zuidex.com. Date accessed: May 25, 2007.

21. Transrectal Ultrasound Scan and Biopsy of the Prostate

Hashim Hashim and Paul Abrams

Indications

Transrectal ultrasound scan (TRUSS) and prostate biopsy (PBx) are mainly used for the diagnosis of prostate cancer (CaP) in patients with elevated prostate-specific antigen (PSA) levels and/or abnormal digital rectal examinations. TRUSS is used to image the prostate and to aid in guiding the biopsy needle. PBx can also be of help in the diagnosis of benign prostatic hyperplasia (BPH) and prostatitis, prostatic abscesses, and prostatic calculi. TRUSS can also be used to guide needles for aspiration of ejaculatory ducts, prostatic cysts, or prostatic abscesses.

TRUSS can be used to determine prostate volume, which will aid in the delivery of treatments such as brachytherapy, and to monitor cryotherapy treatment for CaP. It can also be used in evaluating men with azoospermia to rule out ejaculatory duct cysts, seminal vesicular cysts, müllerian cysts, or utricular cysts.

Contraindications for biopsy include acute painful perianal disorders or a tight anus preventing the probe from being passed, hemorrhagic diatheses, and patients on anticoagulants.

Procedure

1. The procedure should be fully explained to the patient.
2. We suggest giving patients 2 days of 500 mg twice-daily ciprofloxacin (fluoroquinolone) before the procedure. There is some evidence that giving 1 g ciprofloxacin 30 mins before the procedure is sufficient as prophylaxis.
3. We normally give gentamicin (an aminoglycoside) 3 mg/kg intravenously as a prophylactic antibiotic just before the procedure. You will need to discuss the antibiotic prophylaxis with your local microbiologist.
4. Place the patient in the left lateral position with the knees brought up to the chest and the feet pushed away from the body. Other positions that can be used include lithotomy or knee-elbow positions.

5. Perform a digital rectal examination to exclude any masses in the rectum and to feel the prostate, using a topical anesthetic gel/ointment for lubrication.
6. You should be familiar with operating the TRUSS machine (Figure 21.1) before embarking on performing the scanning.
7. Cover the TRUSS endorectal probe (Figure 21.2) with a sterile condom and lubricate it adequately. Depending on the machine you use, some probes require two condoms with gel inserted between the two condoms. The 7-MHz transducer within the endorectal probe, which has a tightly curved array with a wide field of view, is the most

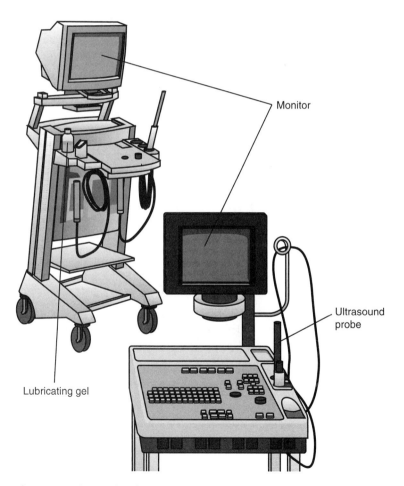

Figure 21.1. Ultrasound Machines.

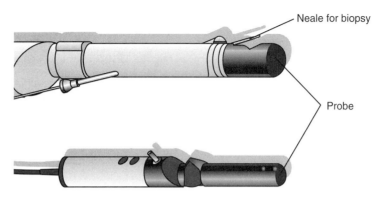

Figure 21.2. Ultrasound Probes.

commonly used transducer. It can produce images in both the sagittal and axial planes.

8. Insert the probe into the rectum gently in the same manner as you would when doing a digital rectal examination (i.e., do not insert it straight into the rectum). Lay the probe flat against the anus and gently slide it into the rectum. Aim initially towards the coccyx and then direct the tip towards the umbilicus.

9. Scan the prostate from apex to base to get a general overview, both in the axial and sagittal views.

10. Find the prostate base and using a 5- or 7-inch 22-gauge spinal needle inserted through the ultrasound probe, inject 5 mL of 1% lidocaine on each side and lateral to the junction of the prostate and the seminal vesicle into the region of the prostatic neurovascular pedicle at the base of the prostate. This provides a periprostatic nerve block. You will be able to observe a "wheal" on TRUSS and see the capsule rising and a triangle forming.

11. Withdraw the needle and move the probe to the apex of the prostute. Inject 2.5 mL of 1% lidocaine into either side at the prostatic apex.

12. Withdraw the needle from the probe.

13. Allow 2 minutes for the anesthetic to work. In the meantime prostate volume can be measured.

14. An alternative local anesthetic technique is the intraprostatic block technique, where 10 mL of 1% lidocaine is injected into two or three sites of each prostate lobe.

15. The examination is made easier if the bladder is slightly filled with urine.

16. The most common method to measure prostate volume requires three measurements of the prostate. The transverse and anteroposterior dimensions are measured (in centimeters) in the axial plane, in the middle portion of the prostate, as this is the widest part. Then the

longitudinal (superior-inferior) diameter is measured (also in centi-meters) in the sagittal plane just off the midline because the bladder neck can obscure the cephalad extent of the gland. Hard-copy images of these are made. The three measurements are used to calculate the volume using the ellipsoid formula: Volume (cm^3) = (anteroposterior [cm]) × (transverse [cm]) × (longitudinal [cm]) × (π/6).

17. Once the volume is calculated, the PSA density (PSA level divided by the prostate volume) can be calculated. If PSA density is greater than 1.5, then this may help in deciding to proceed with a biopsy or not, in some situations.

18. Begin with the axial plane at the base of the prostate to image the prostate and seminal vesicles. The seminal vesicles (convoluted, cystic, and darkly anechoic) are identified bilaterally, with the ampullae of the vas on either side of the midline. Normal seminal vesicle dimensions are 3 cm in length (±0.5 cm), 1.5 cm in width (±0.4 cm), and 13.7 mL in volume (±3.7 mL).

19. Identify the urethra and the verumontanum in the sagittal plane. The level of the verumontanum can be identified by observing the Eiffel tower sign (anterior shadowing) (Figure 21.3).

20. Identify the prostate capsule in the axial plane, which is a hyperechoic (bright compared to normal tissue) structure that can be identified all around the prostate gland.

21. Identify the different zones of the prostate.
   • The transition zone is the central part of the gland and is usually hypoechoic (dark compared to normal tissue) and filled with cystic spaces in patients with BPH.
   • The peripheral zone forms most of the gland volume and is isoechoic. It is usually distal to the verumontanum.

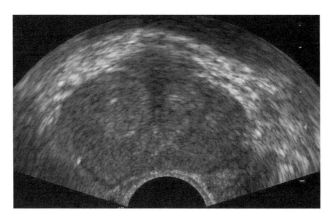

Figure 21.3. Eiffel Tower Sign (Axial View).

- The central zone comprises the posterior part of the gland and is hyperechoic.
- The junction between the peripheral and transition zone is distinct posteriorly and characterized by a hyperechoic region, which results from prostatic calculi or corpora amylacea.
- Prostatic venous plexi are hypoechoic, rounded structures that can be found around the prostate gland.

22. Once the different parts of the prostate are identified, biopsies can be taken. These are best performed using a spring-driven needle core biopsy gun.
23. You need to be familiar with assembling the equipment before starting to biopsy. Make sure that the gun fires before inserting into the patient. You probably need an assistant to help you with loading the gun.
24. Pass the needle (18-gauge with an etched tip and small ridges or pits to make it echogenic) into the gun, through the needle guide attached to the ultrasound probe. The aim is to have prostate biopsy specimens that are 1.5 cm in length.
25. The path of the needle tip during a biopsy is approximately 2.5 cm. The biopsy notch, which enters the tissue, is approximately 1.5 cm. This implies that if you are taking a biopsy of a suspicious lesion, it is important for the needle tip to be placed precisely at the boundary of the lesion before activating the biopsy gun.
26. Some equipment allows you to visualize both sagittal and axial views at the same time and others don't. If your machine does not allow that, then biopsies are taken in the sagittal plane (Figure 21.4). Some people find taking biopsies in the axial view easier.
27. Most equipment allows ultrasound images to be superimposed with a ruled puncture trajectory, in the sagittal plane, that corresponds to the needle guide of the probe, which provides optimal visualization of the biopsy needle path.
28. The number of biopsies taken depends on local protocols. Six biopsies (three from each side) used to be the norm. However, nowadays at least four biopsies need to be taken in small glands and five or six in large glands, from each lobe. This is in addition to biopsies of areas that look suspicious on ultrasound or feel suspicious on digital rectal examination.
29. Three biopsies are obtained from the middle of the prostate in the para-sagittal region at the base, mid-gland, and apex regions. Two further biopsies are taken from the lateral one-third of each lobe near the base and apex. This is done bilaterally, thus totalling ten biopsies. Recent recommendations suggest concentrating on the peripheral zone as this is where most prostate cancer is found, especially on the first set to biopsies.
30. When the biopsies are taken from top to bottom, the probe will need to be moved down to the appropriate area, and you will need to switch between axial and sagittal views to confirm the correct position. You do not need to remove the probe from the rectum. However, the needle

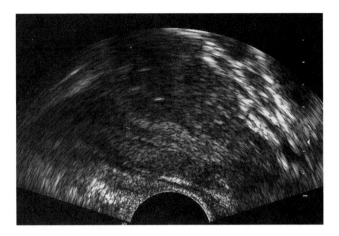

Figure 21.4. Sagittal View of the Prostate.

and gun will need to be removed between biopsies of the different regions so the specimens can be removed and the gun reloaded using the same needle.

31. It is easier to do one lobe first and then do the other lobe as this also avoids confusion. All the biopsies from one lobe can be placed in one specimen pot and the biopsies from the other lobe can be placed in a separate specimen pot. It is important to label the specimen pots correctly and accurately. You can place suspicious areas in a separate pot if you want and label it accurately.

32. Once you finish taking the last biopsy remove the needle and then the probe.

33. Inspect the anus and make sure there isn't profuse bleeding.

34. It is our protocol to insert 400 mg of metronidazole suppository into the rectum at this stage. This also allows us to perform a digital rectal examination and look for bleeding.

35. Give the patient ciprofloxacin 500 mg twice daily orally for 3 days.

36. Send the specimens to the pathology laboratory for histological analysis and arrange appropriate follow-up for the patient.

Complications

Occasional complications include:

• Bleeding from the rectum and urethra (during urination or ejaculation)

- Infection (prostatic and/or urinary tract), requiring hospitalization
- Pain and dull ache in the perineum
- Vasovagal attack during the procedure

Rare complications include:

- High rectal perforation, leading to peritonitis and requiring a laparotomy
- Acute urinary retention, requiring catheterization

References

1. Alavi AS, Soloway MS, Vaidya A, et al. Local anesthesia for ultrasound guided prostate biopsy: a prospective randomized trial comparing 2 methods. J Urol 2001;166(4):1343–1345.
2. Mutaguchi K, Shinohara K, Matsubara A, et al. Local anesthesia during 10 core biopsy of the prostate: comparison of 2 methods. J Urol 2005;173(3):742–745.
3. Pareek G, Armenakas NA, Fracchia JA. Periprostatic nerve blockade for transrectal ultrasound guided biopsy of the prostate: a randomized, double-blind, placebo con-trolled study. J Urol 2001;166(3):894–897.
4. Lee F, Gray JM, McLeary RD, et al. Transrectal ultrasound in the diagnosis of prostate cancer: location, echogenicity, histopathology, and staging. Prostate 1985;7(2): 117–129.
5. Elabbady AA, Khedr MM. Extended 12-core prostate biopsy increases both the detec-tion of prostate cancer and the accuracy of Gleason score. Eur Urol 2006;49(1):49–53; discussion 53.

22. Urodynamics

Christopher Wolter and Roger Dmochowski

Indications

Urodynamic testing is useful in a wide variety of clinical settings in urology. It is useful to confirm or refute clinical suspicion in the general setting of bladder storage and emptying function and dysfunction. The information provided by urodynamics can be very powerful in shaping medical decision-making and surgical management. The scope of this chapter is not to go into the numerous specific indications for urodynamics and the management possibilities of what is found, but to provide technical information on how to set up and perform a good multi-channel urodynamic study. The use of video fluoroscopy will be included, and though it is not universally necessary, it is very useful in certain situations. The steps below will outline how to run a typical urodynamic study, including uroflow, cystometrogram (filling/storage), pressure-flow (emptying), and voiding cystourethrogram (VCUG).

Procedure

1. Obtain informed consent for the procedure.
2. If previous urinalysis or clinical suspicion warrants, check a urine culture at the visit before the procedure. Always check a urinalysis the day of the procedure.
3. Have the patient show up for the procedure with a full bladder. The first phase is an uninstrumented free uroflow. Have the patient void in private as they normally would into a uroflow meter (Figure 22.1).
4. Catheterize the patient for a post-void residual after this.
5. Prior to placing the urodynamic catheters, they need to be set up to the specifications of the urodynamic equipment (Figures 22.2 and 22.3) being used (may need to consult instructions of the machine you are using).
6. Next, place the rectal catheter. Fill balloon of the catheter with recommended amount of fluid (3–5 cc). It is important to remember that the rectal catheters do not have a hole. Thus if you keep on flushing, the balloon continues to expand, resulting in false rectal pressures. It is therefore advisable to make a small cut in the rectal balloon to avoid over-filling (Figure 22.4).

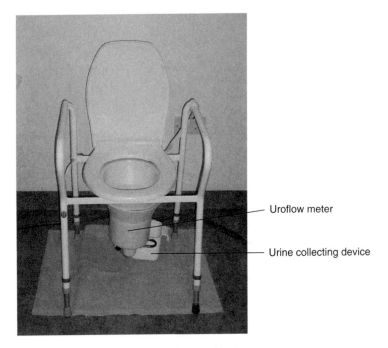

Figure 22.1. Female Flow Meter (Bristol Urological Institute).

7. Place the electromyograph (EMG) electrodes next. For most patients, patch electrodes are sufficient and most comfortable. Needle electrodes are available, but are more invasive and less comfortable. These are more appropriate for patients with decreased sensation, such as those with spinal lesions. The electrodes are placed near the anus over the sphincter at opposite sides of the sphincter (2- to 3 o'clock and 9- to 10 o'clock positions). Ensure the area is clean and free of hair before placing electrodes. Place grounding electrode on thigh (Figure 22.5). This is not universally available and is not a prerequisite for a good urodynamic study.

8. Now, place the urethral catheter. A multi-lumen catheter is typically used (Figure 22.6).

9. Seat the patient on the urodynamic chair or table. Adjust the fluoroscopy source so that the pelvis is in full view (Figure 22.7). Set the pressures so that the vesical and abdominal tracings are equal (this should be a function available on the urodynamic software, but can be adjusted manually). The reference height for all measurements is taken as being level with the upper edge of the symphysis pubis and the transducers are zeroed to atmospheric pressure (Figure 22.8).

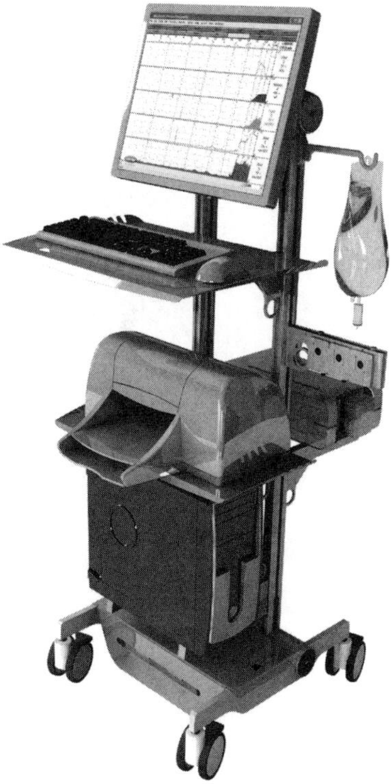

Figure 22.2. Laborie Dorado Urodynamic System (Laborie).

10. Have the patient valsalva and/or cough to ensure the abdominal and vesical tracings are both reading correctly (you should see a definite spike in both tracings).
11. To ensure accurate measurements, the bladder line, rectal line, and all tubing should be flushed to ensure that all air-bubbles have been removed before recording begins. In addition, all connections should be tight, as any leak will cause errors in the pressure measurements recorded. Pressure values will tend to be lower, and recorded with a delay, if there are bubbles or leaks in the pressure system.
12. Begin filling the patient. Typical starting filling rate is 50–60 cc/min. This can be too fast in some instances (for example history or voiding diary suggests low capacity or predominant storage symptoms) or too slow in others (known high post-void residual [PVR] or increased capacity). Proceed accordingly.
13. During filling, especially in symptomatic women, a valsalva leak point pressure will need to be obtained. This is usually done at 150–200 cc,

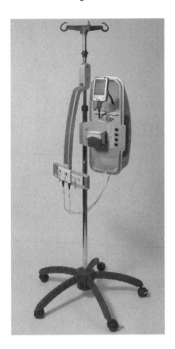

Figure 22.3. World's First Handheld PC Urodynamics Machine (Laborie).

though it can be repeated at a higher volume. Stop filling and have the patient cough and valsalva under live fluoroscopy. Note if there is any leakage, either on fluoroscopy or by directly visualizing the patient's urethra *(1)*.

14. Continue to fill the patient after this. Keep a close eye on the tracing and how it relates to how the patient is relaying their sensation and symptoms to you. Periodically check fluoro images, especially if the

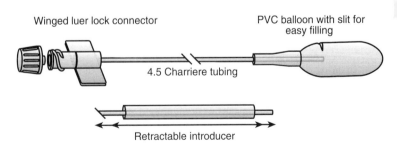

Figure 22.4. Single-Lumen Rectal Catheter With Slit in Balloon (Mediplus).

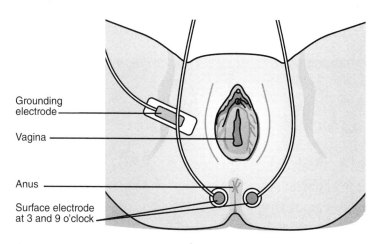

Grounding electrode

Vagina

Anus

Surface electrode at 3 and 9 o'clock

Figure 22.5. EMG Electrodes Placement (Life-tech).

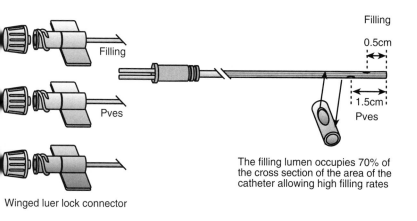

Filling

0.5cm

Filling

Pves

1.5cm

Pves

Winged luer lock connector

The filling lumen occupies 70% of the cross section of the area of the catheter allowing high filling rates

Pves: lumen measuring vesical pressure

Pura: lumen measuring urethral pressure profile

Figure 22.6. Double-Lumen Bladder Catheter, Allowing Simultaneous Filling and Measurement of Vesical Pressure; and Triple-Lumen, Allowing Measurement of Urethral Pressure Profile.

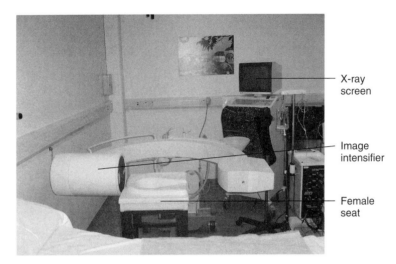

Figure 22.7. Video-Urodynamics Setup for Females Showing Image Intensifier, Seat, and X-ray Screen (Bristol Urological Institute).

patient has symptomatic urges and leakage. If vesicoureteral reflux is suspected, fluoro up higher on the abdomen to investigate this.

15. Quality control at the start of each cystometry is vital, and should be repeated at regular intervals during the test and again at the end of the test to ensure that good pressure transmission is continuing. This is done by asking the patient to cough and seeing an equal rise in the abdominal and vesical line with no rise (or a small biphasic deflection in a fluid-filled system) on the detrusor line.

16. When the patient states they cannot hold any more fluid, stop filling. At this point begin the pressure-flow portion of the study and concomitant VCUG. There should be an indication on the urodynamic tracing that signifies the start of voluntary micturition. Ask the patient to void normally, as they would at home. Encourage them to position themselves as they would normally. They should try and do so with the examiner in the room, but if they need privacy, allow them that. If they can void with you in the room, be at the ready to capture fluoro images as they void for a VCUG.

17. Once the patient has voided to completion, image them again, noting if there is reflux and relatively how well they empty their bladder.

18. If a second study is needed (i.e., repeating the cystometrogram [CMG] with cystocele reduced or slowing the rate to fill the patient to their expected capacity), do this now.

19. After the patient is done voiding for the last time drain the remaining fluid in the bladder, if any, and then the catheters can be removed. Go over the findings with the patient (Figure 22.9), formulating a plan with them.

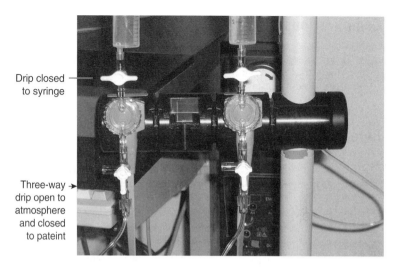

Drip closed to syringe

Three-way drip open to atmosphere and closed to pateint

Figure 22.8. Rectal and Vesical Pressure Transducers (Bristol Urological Institute). Zeroing to atmosphere configuration.

Video image

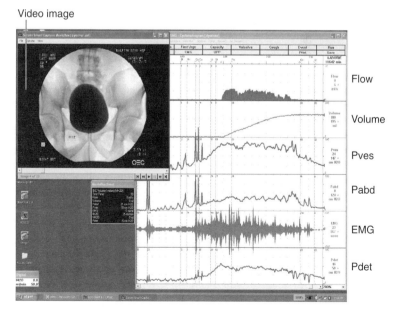

Flow

Volume

Pves

Pabd

EMG

Pdet

Figure 22.9. Video-Urodynamics Screen Image (Laborie).

Complications

- This is a very safe procedure, but complications can be seen
- Urinary tract infection, requiring antibiotics
- Post-procedure irritative symptoms

References

1. Herschorn S, Green J, Robinson D. Videourodynamics. In: *Textbook of Female Urology and Urogynecology*. Cardozo L, Staskin D (Eds). Informa Healthcare; 2006; 301–312.
2. Hashim H, Abrams P. Cystometry. In: *Textbook of Female Urology and Urogynecology*. Cardozo L, Staskin D (Eds). Informa Healthcare; 2006; 225–234.
3. Abrams P, Cardozo L, Fall M, et al. The standardisation of terminology of lower urinary tract function: report form the Standardisation Subcommittee of the International Continence Society. Neurourol Urodyn 2002;21(2):167–178.

23. Flexible Cystoscopy

Christopher Wolter and Roger Dmochowski

Indications

Flexible cystoscopy is now the standard of care for in-office cystoscopy. This is especially true for male patients. This procedure is comfortably and quickly done on the vast majority of patients. The indications for this procedure are the same as for any office cystoscopy, plus the added benefit of being able to perform the procedure with little patient discomfort (1). The typical indications are in investigation for hematuria, follow-up surveillance of transitional cell carcinoma of the bladder, urethroscopy for possible stricture disease of difficult catheterization, ureteral stent removal in office, or any other number of reasons for looking in the bladder.

Procedure

1. The patient should be consented appropriately. They should expect some discomfort. The endoscopist should keep a dialog going with the patient during the procedure to let them know what to expect and what the findings are as the procedure is carried out.
2. Pre-procedure antibiotics can be given, though they are not always necessary.
3. The patient should be placed on the table in the supine position if male and in the low dorsal lithotomy position or "frog-legged" position if female. Alternatively, you can ask the women to bend their knees keeping the feet together and then spreading the knees apart. Once the cystoscope is in the bladder they can straighten their legs but keep them spread apart.
4. An appropriate antiseptic skin and genital prep should be done. Drape accordingly.
5. A viscous lidocaine gel injected intra-urethrally (use approximately 20 mL) before the procedure will aid in patient comfort and provide lubrication for the procedure. A penile clamp can be placed on the male patient to hold the gel in for an appropriate amount of time (2).
6. The flexible cystoscope (Figure 23.1) should have at minimum a light source (Figure 23.2) and irrigation solution (either normal saline or sterile H_2O). An optional endoscope camera and monitor can be used

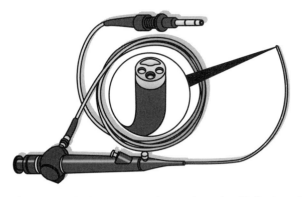

Figure 23.1. Flexible Cystoscope Showing the Angles of Deflection and Field of View.

as well. The patient can be asked if they want to view the procedure on the monitor with you.

7. Familiarize yourself with the flexible cystoscope and its controls. Focus the scope close up before proceeding. It should be held in the dominant hand, with the thumb of that hand on the directional control.

8. With the scope well lubricated and the irrigant running, carefully introduce the scope into the urethral meatus. It should cannulate easily.

9. More so in the male patient, at this point, carefully inspect the urethra. The areas of the fossa navicularis, the penile urethra, and bulbar urethra will be encountered. In males, when reaching the membranous urethra, the external urinary sphincter will be encountered. Here is where the patient may experience some discomfort. Let him know this.

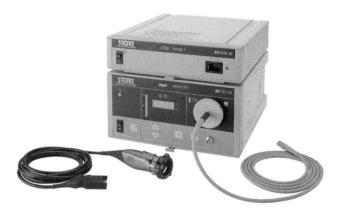

Figure 23.2. Camera and Light Source.

The resistance of this should be easily overcome with the irrigant running and with lubrication. In female patients, advance the scope into the bladder initially.

10. The prostatic urethra should be inspected next. The location of the verumontanum, the relationship of the prostatic lobes, and the height of the bladder neck and medial lobe can be assessed. Advance past this and into the bladder.

11. If the bladder is full, you can turn off the irrigant at this point. Otherwise leave it running if the patient is comfortable. A systematic inspection of the bladder mucosa should be carried out. Deflecting the scope to various degrees, rotate the scope from side to side to completely visualize the bladder. To visualize the ureteral orifices, the scope can be deflected downward and rotated away from the side you are trying to visualize. Upward deflection should be enough to see the dome of the bladder and the air bubble usually introduced by the procedure. Pushing the scope further in and deflecting upward further will actually cause the scope to look back on itself in a retrograde fashion. The bladder neck can be seen in this manner.

12. Once the bladder has been adequately inspected, if needed, instruments can be introduced for various tasks such as ureteral stent removal, biopsy of the bladder, or guidewire placement for difficult catheterization.

13. Once cystoscopy is complete, the irrigant should be turned on again and urethroscopy should be repeated, or in the case of the female patient it can be performed now. Slowly and carefully withdraw the scope while doing this.

14. The findings can be shared and summarized with the patient at this point.

15. Ensure the patient is able to void after the procedure if doing so normally before.

Complications

- Minor hematuria, which is usually self-limiting
- Infection, requiring antibiotics
- Irritative voiding symptoms, which are usually self-limiting
- Rarely, perforation of the bladder if other instruments are introduced. This can be treated with in-dwelling catheterization in most cases.

References

1. Pavone-Macaluso M, Lamartina M, Pavone C, Vella M. The flexible cystoscope. Int Urol Nephrol 1992;24(3):239–242.
2. Selman SH. Endoscopy and instrumentation in the office. In: *Office Urology*. Kursh ED, Ulchaker JC (Eds). Totowa: Humana; 2001; 89–101.

24. Rigid Cystoscopy

Christopher Wolter and Roger Dmochowski

Indications

Rigid cystoscopy is at the very core of a large portion of the urologists' armamentarium. It can provide access to the lower and upper urinary tract, and can be used for diagnostic purposes as well as numerous adjunctive therapeutic procedures, so many that it exceeds the scope of this chapter. Furthermore, cystoscopy is ubiquitous throughout all sub-specialties in the field of urology, whether it is for the pediatric patient, the oncology patient, or the patient with kidney stones. For the purposes of this chapter, we will focus on the basics of rigid cystoscopy and its technical aspects.

Procedure

1. Obtain informed consent for the procedure.
2. General anesthesia is usually chosen, though rigid cystoscopy can be comfortably done on women in a clinic setting with them awake (1).
3. Preoperative antibiotics are normally given.
4. Place the patient on a cystoscopy table in the lithotomy position. Be careful in positioning, ensuring the patient is properly padded and that the hands and fingers are away from the table break. Do not overly rotate the patient's hips (2).
5. Prep the skin of the genital area with an aqueous betadine or chlorhexidine solution. Drape the field accordingly.
6. Familiarize yourself with the equipment. There should be at least a 21-F sheath, a working bridge, and Albarran bridge if instrumentation is planned, a 0° or 12° lens, a 30° lens, and a 70° lens (Figures 24.1 and 24.2). A light source and irrigant (e.g., 0.9% normal saline or 5% glucose), appropriate for the procedure are also necessary. A camera and monitor are very helpful, though optional (Figure 24.3).
7. In males begin by inserting the lubricated scope with a 0°, 12° or 30° lens in order to visualize the urethral lumen so that it can be navigated atraumatically. For women, especially if they are awake, it may be more advantageous to begin by inserting the sheath with a blunt obturator in (Figure 24.4).

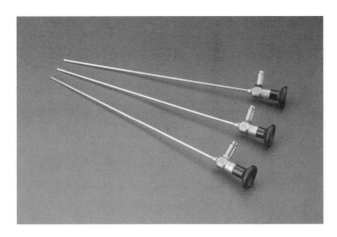

Figure 24.1. Rigid Cystoscopes With Different Viewing Angles.

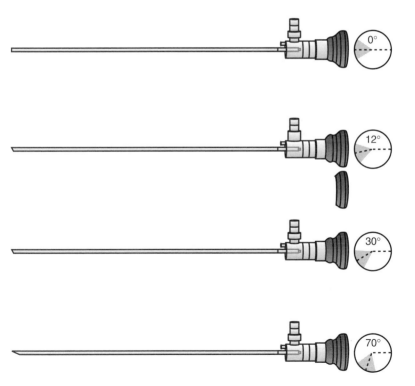

Figure 24.2. Schematic Diagram of Different Viewing Angles Cystoscopes.

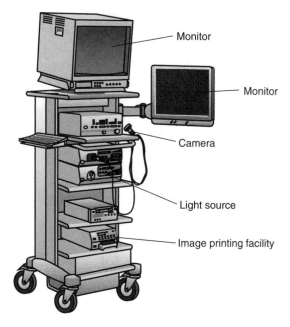

Figure 24.3. Monitor and Light Stack.

8. Once the urethra has been traveled and the bladder entered, drain the bladder. Refill with irrigant. Systematically inspect the bladder and ureteral orifices. This will require manipulating the scope and rotating it to use the benefit of the angle of the lens in place.

9. Make note of the quality and character of the bladder mucosa and underlying structure if appreciated. Are there masses, erythematous patches, trabeculations, or diverticula present?

10. Be sure to use the 70° lens in order to completely and confidently inspect the entire bladder, especially the anterior, dome and lateral surfaces. Using the 70° lens on awake females will also reduce the angulation needed to completely visualize the bladder, thus reducing discomfort.

11. If being performed, proceed with any adjunctive procedures at this time.

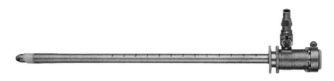

Figure 24.4. Sheath and Blunt Obturator.

12. When you have confidently inspected the bladder completely, drain it, then open the irrigant port and withdraw the scope into the urethra. Carefully perform urethroscopy on the way out, removing all components of the scope at this time.

Complications

- Hematuria, usually mild and self-limiting
- Infection, requiring antibiotics
- Dysuria or urethral discomfort
- Damage to or perforation of the bladder, requiring prolonged catheterization or surgical repair
- Damage to the bladder related to additional procedures performed in the same setting
- Urethral stricture

References

1. Selman SH. Endoscopy and instrumentation in the office. In: *Office Urology*. Kursh ED, Ulchaker JC (Eds). Totowa: Humana; 2001;89–101.
2. McEwen DR. Intraoperative positioning of surgical patients. AORN J 1996; 63(6):1059–1079.

25. Suprapubic Catheterization

Christopher Wolter and Roger Dmochowski

Indications

Suprapubic catheterization is a very useful procedure that is indicated in a variety of settings. Generally speaking, it is a way to provide bladder drainage when urethral access is not possible or advisable or by itself is insufficient. This could present in a number of scenarios. Urethral disruption, severe urethral stricture disease, or an inaccessible urethra owing to traumatic catheterization are possible indications. Additionally, when maximal bladder drainage is desired in the post-operative setting, such as after major repair, a suprapubic catheter is indicated. This can also be the case after urethral repair when a precautionary alternative drainage is desirable once the urethral catheter is removed. Finally, it can be an alternative to chronic in-dwelling urethral catheterization, as it is generally easier to take care of and considered more sanitary. Here we will discuss the technique of placing a suprapubic catheter and the various clinical scenarios it can be encountered.

Procedure

In the Setting Where Urethral Access Is Inadvisable or Not Available (1)

1. Obtain the proper consent for the procedure. This should be done under general anesthesia.
2. Pre-operative antibiotics should be given. Choose one with good urinary concentration (e.g., fluoroquinolones).
3. Prep the lower abdomen and genitalia with aqueous betadine or chlorhexidine.
4. Consider whether the patient has had previous abdominal surgeries. If so, proceed with caution. You can position the patient in the Trendelenburg position to help move the bowel away from the bladder.
5. Make a small vertical incision (4–5 cm) in the midline, starting from the pubic symphysis and going up.
6. Using electrocautery, dissect through the subcutaneous fat and Scarpa's fascia. Expose the rectus fascia.

7. Using sharp dissection or cautery, open the rectus fascia. This can be done in either the vertical or horizontal direction.
8. Without dividing the muscle, retract the rectus muscle bellies from the midline. This should expose the underlying transversalis fascia and bladder immediately beneath this.
9. Ideally, the bladder will be full. If you are unsure, you can insert a small-gauge needle attached to a syringe to confirm the bladder is in the operative field.
10. Next, place vertical stay sutures or 3/0 synthetic absorbable sutures on either side of midline. You can also grab the bladder with Allis clamps in a similar fashion.
11. Using the cut current or with a scalpel, open the bladder. Keep the cystotomy small.
12. Insert a catheter into the cystotomy. If using a Malecot-tip catheter, straighten the phlanges over a clamp. A balloon catheter can be inserted as well. Inflate the balloon.
13. When the catheter is in, ensure that it is not placed too far in, and that it is not touching the trigone or bladder neck.
14. Close the cystotomy now with either interrupted 3/0 synthetic absorbable sutures or with a purse-string closure.
15. Make a small incision in the skin and bring the catheter out through this incision, passing a clamp through the incision and the fascia to bring it out. Secure to the skin with a drain stitch.
16. Close the fascia. A drain can be placed if desired. Close the skin and subcutaneous tissues in separate layers.

In the Setting Where Urethral Access Is Available

1. This version of the procedure is preferable if the procedure is elective, the urethra is accessible, and the patient has had no previous lower abdominal procedures.
2. Pass a curved Lowsley retractor or sound with an eye at the tip through the urethra and into the bladder.
3. Angle the instrument so the tip points upward and can be palpated through the bladder and abdominal wall immediately above the pubic symphysis.
4. Cut down directly onto the instrument with the cut current or a scalpel. Keep the upward traction on the instrument, and it should come out suprapubicly after the incision is made.
5. Either grasp a catheter in the jaws of the Lowsley retractor or loop a suture through the hole in the catheter and the Lowsley or sound.
6. Pull the instrument back into the bladder and out through the urethra. Carefully withdraw the tip of the catheter back into the lumen of the bladder. Inflate the balloon and retract the catheter to the dome of the bladder. Confirm good positioning with cystoscopy.
7. Secure the catheter to the patient.

Using a Percutaneous Kit

1. This is advisable in patients with a full bladder (can be confirmed by ultrasonography). It is highly preferable that they have had no previous abdominal procedures. This technique can be done easily under local anesthesia. Make sure to inject the local anesthetic deep enough to anesthetize the fascia.

2. Advance a 20-guage spinal needle through the skin and into the bladder. You should only need to angle the needle about 10–15°, from the vertical position, so that it is pointing slightly towards the foot. Advance until urine is aspirated. This will confirm the location of the bladder by direction and depth.

3. Make a 1-cm transverse incision in the midline approximately 2 cm (two fingerbreadths) above the pubic symphysis, through the site where you inserted the needle.

4. The next step depends on the kit being used. You should advance the trocar and sheath in the same direction and depth as you did with the locating needle. Once in the bladder, urine should come out from the sheath. You normally feel a give in the trocar once the fascia is pierced.

5. Push slightly further into the bladder and remove the trocar. Cover the tip of the sheath so that urine does not rush out.

6. Insert the catheter through the sheath and inflate the catheter balloon with the specified volume of sterile water, as indicated on the catheter.

7. Remove the peel-away sheath and pull the catheter back until resistance is met, indicating the catheter is sitting on the bladder wall.

8. Attach the catheter to a urine meter drainage bag.

9. Secure the catheter to the patient with a synthetic non-absorbable suture, if needed. If available, you can confirm placement with cystoscopy or, alternatively, perform the whole procedure under cystoscopic guidance.

Complications

- Bleeding
- Infection, requiring antibiotics
- Dislodgment of the catheter
- Obstruction or clogging of the catheter with debris
- Encrustation with stones
- Perforation of the bowel or other intra-abdominal structures, requiring repair and/or bowel diversion
- Bladder spasm or discomfort from the catheter being advanced too far in the bladder

- Urine leak after catheter removal. This is usually self-limiting, though it may require urethral catheter drainage to resolve completely.

Reference

1. Suprapubic catheterization. In: *Atlas of Urologic Surgery, 2nd Edition.* Hinman F Jr (Ed). Philadelphia: Saunders; 1998;625–629.

26. Cystodiathermy

Christopher Wolter and Roger Dmochowski

Indications

Cystodiathermy is a useful procedure for small lesions of the bladder, or for obtaining hemostasis after biopsy of the bladder. It is performed by using a high-frequency electrode to essentially cauterize select areas of the bladder. If used for bladder tumors, ensure that they are small and superficial, as larger tumors generally require a deeper resection. It is a procedure that requires minimal anesthesia and is overall tolerated well by patients. Standard rigid or flexible cystoscopy can be employed for this procedure. Rigid cystoscopy usually requires a deeper level of anesthesia, whereas flexible cystoscopy can even be done on the awake patient and is tolerated relatively well, though it can be technically more challenging (1).

Procedure

1. Obtain consent for the procedure.
2. Set up the patient as for the method of cystoscopy you are using (*see* Chapters 23 and 24).
3. In addition to the cystoscopy setup, an electrical dispersion pad connected to the energy source should be placed on the patient, and the fluid used for the procedure should be sterile water of a 1.5% glycine solution. A foot pedal for the energy source is also necessary and should be placed in a location that is easily accessible to the surgeon.
4. Preoperative antibiotics can be used, if necessary.
5. If performing the procedure with flexible cystoscopy, use intra-urethral lidocaine jelly, and a lidocaine solution can be instilled into the bladder as well for additional comfort. If performing using rigid cystoscopy, general anesthesia or closely monitored anesthesia care should be employed.
6. Proceed with cystoscopy. Once in the bladder, completely visualize the entire lumen before proceeding. If the amount of disease is greater than anticipated, consider proceeding with a formal transurethral resection and fulguration.
7. Center the scope view on the lesion. Advance the electrode through the working port of the scope, if using flexible cystoscope, and advance

until it is seen in bladder. If using a rigid cystoscope you will need a 30° scope and an Albarran bridge to direct the electrode. Some centers use lasers instead of electrocautery, but this requires specialized equipment.

8. Keep the tip of the electrode a safe distance from the lens. Have the circulating nurse set the power on the device to an appropriate level (generally a setting of 30–50 on most generators).

9. Touch the base of the lesion with the tip of the electrode. Push the pedal and cauterize the lesion. If the lesion takes more than one treatment, as most will, move the electrode accordingly and treat again. It is advisable to treat an area that is 20–25% larger than the original lesion in order to ensure there is no residual tumor remaining. Take care not to over-treat in one area as far as depth is concerned.

10. If treating a bleeding area, such as after a biopsy, place the tip of the electrode directly on the bleeding surface or vessel and cauterize. It may be necessary to treat wider than the bleeding area to get it to stop completely, but avoid this if possible. Again, be mindful of the depth you are treating.

11. Drain the bladder and visualize the area treated again after refilling. Observe for several seconds to ensure that the lesion is completely treated and that the bleeding has stopped.

12. Treat all other areas as needed.

13. Place a Foley catheter if clinically warranted. This can generally be discontinued in the recovery area or on post-op Day 1 if desired.

Complications

- Bleeding, possibly requiring a second procedure
- Infection, requiring antibiotics
- Pain during or after the procedure
- Bladder spasm or irritation post-procedure
- Rarely, perforation of the bladder, requiring prolonged catheterization or additional surgery
- Recurrence of the lesion treated

Reference

1. Wedderburn AW, Ratan P, Birch BR. A prospective trial of flexible cystodiathermy for recurrent transitional cell carcinoma of the bladder. J Urol 1999;161(3):812–814.

27. Cystodistension (Hydrodistension)

Hashim Hashim and Paul Abrams

Indications

Hydrodistension is mainly indicated for the diagnosis and/or treatment of painful bladder syndrome (interstitial cystitis), although there is there is no guarantee that it will relieve bladder symptoms. There are no clear guidelines on how this procedure should be performed and below is one recommendation of how it could be done.

Procedure

1. Place the patient in the supine position on the operating table and place the legs in the lithotomy position.
2. Perform a digital rectal examination in men or a vaginal examination in women to assess the presence of any masses.
3. Clean the perineal region with chlorhexidine and drape accordingly.
4. Insert a 0° (or 12°) lens to perform urethroscopy and then cystoscopy in the bladder (*see* Chapters 23 and 24).
5. Empty the bladder to measure "residual urine" and therefore bladder capacity by removing the cystoscope but keeping the sheath in the bladder.
6. Re-insert a 70° cystoscope.
7. Have a look around the bladder for any pathology (e.g., Hunners ulcers)
8. Fill the bladder with saline through the cystoscope with the fluid level in the irrigation bag 30 cm above the symphisis pubis.
9. Make sure you close the outflow of the cystoscope when filling the bladder.
10. Measure maximum bladder capacity. This is reached when:
    - There is cessation of fluid inflow
    - There is blanching of vessels
    - The patient becomes "restless" under general anesthesia with raised pulse rate and blood pressure
11. Empty the bladder, measure the bladder capacity, and elevate the fluid bag to 100 cm above the symphisis pubis.

12. Commence slow filling of the bladder. Do not distend beyond a capacity of 1,000 mL.
13. Distend for 1 minute and then empty the bladder and record the capacity.
14. Observe for glomerulations.
15. Repeat the distension procedure a maximum of five times, or until there is no further increase in the volume of the distended bladder. Alternatively, distend the bladder, only once, for 10 minutes, by leaving a catheter with an inflated balloon, in site.
16. Re-measure the bladder capacity again by filling the bladder through the cystoscope with the fluid level lying 30 cm above the symphisis pubis.
17. Record the bladder volumes in a standard fashion:
    - Initial capacity at 30 cm water pressure
    - Maximum distension capacity at 100 cm water pressure
    - Final capacity at 30 cm water pressure

Complications

Occasional complications include:

- Mild burning or bleeding on passing urine for short period after operation
- May need temporary insertion of a catheter
- Often a biopsy of the bladder may be performed after distension

Rare complications include:

- Infection of bladder, requiring antibiotics
- Delayed bleeding, requiring removal of clots or further surgery
- Perforation of the bladder, requiring a temporary urinary catheter or return to theater for open surgical repair, if the rupture is intraperitoneal (as shown by cystography)

References

1. Turner KJ, Stewart LH. How do you stretch a bladder? A survey of UK practice, a literature review, and a recommendation of a standard approach. Neurourol Urodyn 2005;24(1):74–76.
2. The British Association of Urological Surgeons (Consent forms). http://www.baus.org.uk. Date accessed: May 25, 2007.

28. Extracorporeal Shockwave Lithotripsy (ESWL)

Christopher Wolter and Roger Dmochowski

Indications

ESWL has proven over time to be a major breakthrough in urology. It is the procedure by which shockwaves are generated at a point external to the body (F1 point) and are focused on a kidney stone in the body (F2 point) (Figure 28.1). The shockwaves themselves are relatively weak at their source and can thus traverse the body without any untoward effects. However, at the point at which they are focused, they are sufficiently powerful to fragment a kidney stone. This is guided by fluoroscopy in most instances, though ultrasound-guided techniques have been described. Fragmenting almost any stone can be attempted with this technique, but the success varies greatly depending on the size and location of the stone. Generally speaking, for stones in the upper and interpolar calyces, and the renal pelvis, the size limit is 2 cm, and for stones in the lower pole, the size limit is 1 cm. Most stones in the upper ureter can be fragmented as well. The larger the stone, the higher the likelihood there will be a need for a second procedure. Contraindications to this procedure include active urinary tract infection, uncontrolled bleeding diathesis, poorly controlled hypertension, and pregnancy. Relative considerations that may prohibit use of ESWL are obesity, deformity of body habitus, suspected anatomic obstruction, stones in a calyceal diverticulum, and renal failure.

Procedure

1. Obtain consent for the procedure, ensuring that the listed complications below are discussed and the side to be treated is marked.
2. Prior to the procedure, obtain a urine culture. Even if the culture is negative, some doctors contemplate using pre-operative antibiotics. Choose an antibiotic that achieves good levels in urine, (i.e., a fluoroquinolone).
3. Depending on the type of machine being used, the anesthesia/analegesia chosen can vary. For the older-generation machines (e.g., Dornier HM3), general anesthesia is necessary. For newer, lower-powered machines (Figure 28.2), simple analgesia, sedation, or monitored anesthetic care can be used.

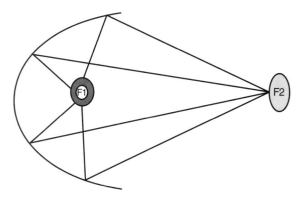

Figure 28.1. F1 and F2 Points.

4. If necessary, a ureteral stent can be placed pre-operatively, either at the same setting or at an earlier date.
5. Place the patient on the ESWL table in the supine position. If using a HM3 lithotriptor, the patient will need to be placed in the harness. Position the patient correctly over the shockwave generator. This may vary depending on the model being used.

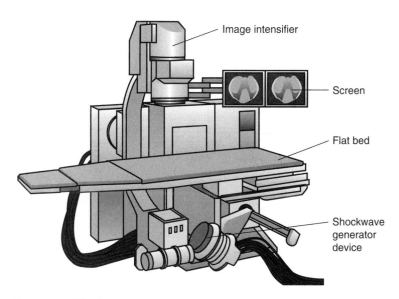

Figure 28.2. Lithotripter.

6. Using the fluoroscopy of the unit, center the stone on the F2 point. Two images taken at 90° from each other are used. This allows the patient to be moved so that the stone is directly at the F2 point.

7. Begin fragmenting the stone. Power settings used are generally recommended for each machine being used. Start at a rate of 120 shocks/minute. Slower rates (80–90), however, can be more effective.

8. The urologist and the anesthesiologist should observe the cardiac monitor closely in this early period. The shockwaves can induce an arrhythmia. If this happens, all is not lost. The shockwave rate needs to be adjusted so that it is coupled to the R-wave on the cardiac monitor. The connection for this should be available with the lithotripter. Proceed again, carefully observing the monitor for additional changes.

9. Every few hundred shocks, the stone should be re-imaged in two directions again. If the patient or the stone has moved, readjust the position of the F2 point by moving the patient. Generally, how often you choose to re-image is up to your discretion. Factors that may contribute to this decision include how many stones there are, how deep under anesthesia the patient is, and the relative amount of free space there is around the stone in the kidney.

10. Continue to shock the stone after the patient has been moved. A total of 2000–2400 shocks are allowed, depending on the machine being used.

11. Once you are finished delivering the shockwaves, take fluoroscopy images once again to see if there are any remaining stone fragments.

12. The patient can go home the same day if stable in recovery. Postoperatively, a short course of antibiotics is recommended. Oral analgesics should be provided as well.

13. Additionally, provide the patient a filter for their urine to collect any stone fragments that may pass so that they can be analyzed.

14. When seeing the patient in follow-up, always repeat imaging to ensure the stone is gone. CT is most sensitive, but plain films or an intravenous urogram can be obtained as well with good confidence.

Complications

- Residual stone fragments
- Steinstrasse or a column of stone fragments trapped behind a larger, obstructing lead fragment in the ureter
- Bleeding into and around the kidney, possibly requiring transfusion (though gross hematuria occurs in most patients)
- Infection, even in the face of a negative urine culture, as the stone could harbor bacteria
- Hypertension

- Transient decrease in renal function, though more lasting in rare instances
- Post-procedure pain

References

1. Lingeman JE, Lifshitz DA, Evan AP. Surgical management of urinary lithiasis. In: *Campbell's Urology, 8th Edition.* Walsh PC (Ed). Philadelphia: Saunders; 2002; 3361–3452.
2. Conlin MJ. Complications of extracorporeal shockwave lithotripsy. In: *Complications of Urologic Surgery.* Taneja SS, Smith RB, Ehrlich RM (Eds). Philadelphia: Saunders; 2001;155–164.

29. Insertion of Double-J Stent

Christopher Wolter and Roger Dmochowski

Indications

This common procedure is indicated in a variety of settings in urology. Its general indication is to relieve obstruction of the ureter. This can be caused by a variety of conditions. Obstruction by a calculus, ureteral stricture, extrinsic compression, and ureteropelvic junction obstruction are just a sample of the conditions this procedure can be employed in. In addition, double-J stents (Figure 29.1) can be placed before other pelvic surgeries to aid in identifying the ureter, though simple ureteral catheters can be used for this as well. Finally, double-J stents can be placed after other reconstructive urologic procedures such as ureteral reimplant, pyeloplasty, or partial nephrectomy. Here we will describe the basic technique employed in placing the double-J stent (double pigtail ended stent on both ends).

Procedure

1. Obtain consent for the procedure and make sure you document the correct side of the operation. If the stent is an adjunctive procedure to a larger surgical procedure, make sure the patient is aware they may leave the operating room with a stent in place.
2. Obtain preoperative urine cultures if this is an elective procedure. If this is an emergent procedure, a culture is not necessary, especially because the stent may be employed to drain an infected collecting system. In any setting, use pre-operative antibiotics.
3. Set up the patient as you would for rigid cystoscopy (*see* Chapter 24).
4. Fluoroscopy is a must to ensure correct and safe positioning, so perform the procedure on a radiolucent table and have a fluoroscopy source in the room.
5. Proceed as you normally would for cystoscopy.
6. Once you are in the bladder, identify the ureter you wish to stent. If clinically indicated, or if you wish to gain better anatomical detail, perform a retrograde pyelogram (*see* Chapter 30) at this time.
7. Pass a flexible-tipped guidewire through the working channel of the Albarran bridge/cystoscope and into the ureteral orifice. If there is

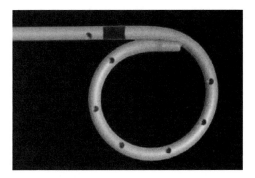

Figure 29.1. One End of a Double-J Stent With Black Mark.

difficulty manipulating the wire, you may want to pass a ureteral catheter through the working channel first.

8. Under fluoroscopic guidance, advance the wire up into the kidney. Be sure to be using the fluoroscopy the entire way in real time. Once the wire coils up in the kidney, you have advanced far enough.

9. If an obstruction is encountered, be very gentle with the wire, as you do not want to create a false passage in the ureter. Advancing the ureteral catheter up the wire can enable greater control over the wire for traction and manipulation. In addition, the wire can then be removed and retrograde pyelography can be performed exactly at the site of obstruction without losing any ground already gained. Alternatively, you can use an ureteroscope to have a look in the obstructed area and help maneuver the guide wire.

10. Once the wire is in the kidney, remove the ureteral catheter. Ensure the guidewire stays in place by performing this task under live fluoroscopy.

11. Select an appropriate-sized stent for the patient's height (5- to 8-F; 20- to 28-cm length). Usually a 6-F 24-cm stent is used in people of average height and 6-F 26-cm in taller people.

12. Advance the double-J stent over the guidewire. Be sure to put the more tapered end first. To aid in orientation, there should also be a black line just before the distal curl (Figure 29.1). Once the stent is pushed into the scope, place the stent pusher over the wire, or use a ureteral catheter to push the stent.

13. While advancing, watch the stent periodically under live fluoroscopy. Once the tip of the stent is in the renal pelvis, watch the cystoscopic image of the stent closely so that it is not advanced too far.

14. When the black line before the distal curl is at the ureteral orifice, back up the scope's view to the level of the bladder neck while keeping the ureteral orifice centered on the screen. Continue to advance now until the tip of the stent pusher is just into view.

15. Under live fluoroscopy, view the stent in the kidney. Slowly withdraw the guidewire. The proximal stent should curl up. Continue to withdraw the wire until it is completely removed. You should see the distal end of the stent curl in your cystoscopic image.
16. Observe the end of the stent for urine drainage.
17. Drain the bladder and remove the equipment from the bladder.
18. You may consider catheterizing the patient if they had ureteric obstruction.

Complications

- Hematuria
- Bladder irritation
- Infection, requiring antibiotics
- Flank pain caused by acute reflux of urine into the kidney
- Proximal or distal migration of the stent that could necessitate other procedures or result in inadequate drainage of the collecting system
- Perforation of ureter during guide are insertion.

Reference

1.   The British Association of Urological Surgeons (Consent form). http://www.baus. org.uk. Date accessed: May 25, 2006.

30. Retrograde Pyelography

Hashim Hashim and Paul Abrams

Indications

Retrograde pyelography involves taking X-rays of the kidney and ureter by injection of contrast through a ureteric stent. This is done mainly for diagnostic indications, including diagnosis of the level of ureteric obstruction and looking for intrinsic lesions of the ureter and kidney that were not very clear on intravenous pyelography.

Procedure

1. Patients need pre-operative counselling regarding the procedure. You will also need to obtain consent for permission for endoscopic removal or biopsy of bladder abnormality or stone if found.
2. The procedure is done under general anesthesia.
3. The patient is placed on an operating table, which allows X-rays to be taken using an image intensifier, which needs to be available in the operating room.
4. Make sure that the side to be operated on is correctly marked.
5. Spread the legs apart by approximately 60°. Place the patient in a position so that the hips are raised approximately 20–30° from the horizontal position, and then bend the knees so that they make an angle of 150° with the thighs (Figure 30.1) (i.e., relatively flat rather than a full lithotomy [modified Lloyd-Davies]). This position helps keep the ureter relatively straight.
6. Administer antibiotics (e.g., gentamicin 3 mg/kg intravenously), if there is suspicion of sepsis.
7. Perform rigid cystoscopy using a 0° or 12° scope (*see* Chapters 23 and 24) to identify the ureteric orifices and inspect the bladder.
8. Remove the telescope, keeping the sheath in the bladder.
9. Use a 70° scope with an Albarran bridge (Figure 30.2) to allow passage of a guidewire.
10. Make sure that the bridge is in the neutral position, and not deflected downwards, as it may cause trauma to the bladder neck. Insert the scope and bridge through the sheath and into the bladder and secure it in place.

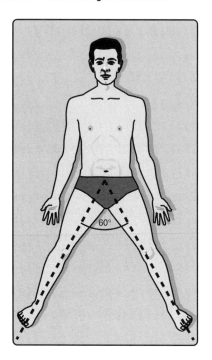

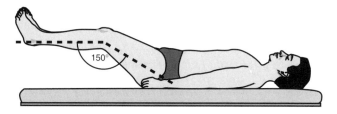

Figure 30.1. Positioning of the Patient's Lower Limbs.

11. Insert an open-ended (Figure 30.3) ureteric catheter or a cone-tip–ended (Figure 30.4) catheter through one of the holes in the Albarran bridge into the correct ureteric orifice. The ureteric catheter normally has a guidewire inside that aids insertion into the ureteric orifice.

12. Once in the ureteric orifice, remove the guidewire and attach a Luer lock (Figure 30.5) onto the ureteric catheter.

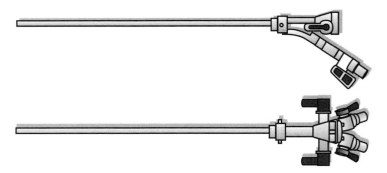

Figure 30.2. Two-Way Albarran Bridge.

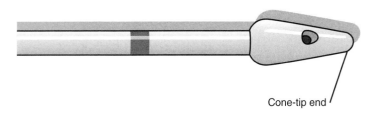

Open end

Figure 30.3. Open-Ended Ureteral Catheter.

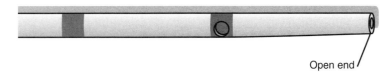

Cone-tip end

Figure 30.4. Cone-Tip – Ended Ureteral Catheter.

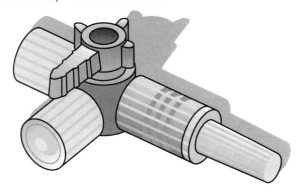

Figure 30.5. Three-Way Luer Lock.

13. Push the ureteric catheter up to the level you suspect there is a problem, under fluoroscopic guidance.
14. Ask your assistant to withdraw 20 mL of iodinated contrast material (e.g., Urografin) into a syringe and attach the syringe to the Luer lock. Hold the syringe upside-down so that the plunger is on the top end. This allows any air bubbles to rise to the top of the syringe and avoids them entering the system and producing artifacts.
15. Instill the contrast material slowly and use simultaneous fluoroscopy to delineate the required anatomy. If you instill the contrast quickly, it may push a possible stone upwards towards the kidney.
16. Once you finished the retrograde, pull the catheter from the ureter and bladder.
17. Remove the cystoscope and sheath from the bladder.

Complications

Common complications include:

- The need for the temporary insertion of a urinary catheter after the procedure
- Use of X-ray imaging to take pictures of urinary tract, which produce radiation
- Failure to insert the ureteric catheter, requiring alternative investigations (e.g., antegrade ureteropyelography)

Rare complications include:

- Infection of the bladder, requiring antibiotics
- Kidney damage or infection, requiring further treatment
- Finding bladder cancer, requiring additional therapy
- Damage to the ureter, which necessitates an open operation or the insertion of a nephrostomy tube antegradely from the back to allow any leak to heal
- Scarring or stricture of the ureter, requiring further procedures
- Allergic reaction to contrast material

Reference

1. The British Association of Urological Surgeons (Consent forms). http://www.baus.org.uk. Date accessed: May 25, 2007.

31. Ureteroscopy (Semi-Rigid)

Hashim Hashim and Paul Abrams

Indications

Ureteroscopy is the passage of a ureteroscope into the ureter. This can be either diagnostic or therapeutic. The diagnostic indications include obstruction of the ureter, intra-luminal lesions, hematuria, abnormal cytology, suspected neoplasm, and surveillance. The therapeutic indications include relief of obstruction, removal of calculi, insertion of stents, treatment of neoplasms, and strictures.

Procedure

1. Patients will need pre-operative counseling regarding the procedure and the possible need for a stent at the time of ureteroscopy. You will also need to obtain consent.
2. Make sure that the side to be operated on is correctly marked.
3. The procedure is done under general anesthesia.
4. The patient is placed on an operating table, which allows X-rays to be taken, as an image intensifier needs to be available in the operating room.
5. Spread the legs apart by approximately 60°. Place the patient in a position so that the hips are raised approximately 20–30° from the horizontal position and then bend the knees so that they make an angle of 150° with the thighs (*see* Figure 30.1) (i.e., relatively flat rather than a full lithotomy [modified Lloyd-Davies]). This position helps keep the ureter relatively straight.
6. Administer antibiotics (e.g., gentamicin 3 mg/kg intravenously) if there is suspicion of sepsis.
7. Perform rigid cystoscopy (*see* Chapter 24) to identify the ureteric orifices and inspect the bladder.
8. Remove the cystoscope but keep the sheath in the bladder.
9. Use a 70° scope with an Albarran bridge (*see* Figure 30.2) attached, to allow passage of a guidewire.
10. Insert the scope and bridge through the sheath and into the bladder, and secure it in place. Make sure that the bridge is up and not deflected downwards.

11. Under fluoroscopic guidance, insert a guidewire through one of the holes in the Albarran bridge into the correct ureteric orifice.
12. Pass the guidewire all the way up to the renal pelvis. This is the "safety" wire. You can use X-ray imaging to confirm position of the guidewire.
13. Remove the cystoscope and sheath together. Make sure that you do not pull the guidewire out as well. It may be easier to remove the cystoscope and bridge first, holding the wire in place inside the sheath, and then remove the sheath.
14. Now insert the ureteroscope (Figure 31.1), under endoscopic camera guidance down the urethra into the bladder. This passage is aided by visualizing the guidewire and following it. You may also need to apply mild hydrostatic pressure to the irrigating fluid to open up the urethra.
15. Now identify the ureteric orifice and insert another guidewire down the working channel of the ureteroscope.
16. Insert the second guidewire 3–4 cm up into the ureter. Confirm the position with the image intensifier.
17. Rotate the ureteroscope 180° and apply mild hydrostatic pressure through the irrigating channel, and then gently pass the ureteroscope into the ureteric orifice. These maneuvers aid insertion into the orifice.
18. Rotate the scope back into the zero initial starting position and visualize the distal ureter. Keep the second guidewire in the original position.
19. Pass the ureteroscope gently up the ureter. You can use the image intensifier to confirm your position.
20. You may find difficulty negotiating the scope up the ureter at the level of the pelvic brim where the iliac vessels cross. It is important not to

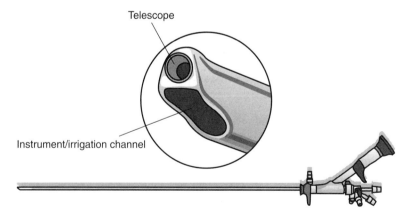

Telescope

Instrument/irrigation channel

Figure 31.1. Semi-Rigid Ureteroscope.

use force with the scope, as it can cause perforation or damage the instrument.

21. Some techniques available to help you pass the scope include:
    - Fill the bladder more, to straighten the intra-mural ureter. However, avoid over-distension of the ureter, as this will kink the ureter.
    - Placing one of your hands on the abdomen at the level of the pelvic brim to try to maneuver the ureteroscope through the abdominal wall.
    - Ask an assistant to elevate the loin on the side.
    - Pass the second guidewire up the ureter over the pelvic brim into the renal pelvis. Then advance the scope also under fluoroscopic guidance over the guidewire (over-wire technique).
    - Use a saline-filled syringe to irrigate through the ureteroscope to open the ureter under pressure. This performs the function of foot pedals which are available in same artery for irrigation.

22. Once the pelvic-brim is passed, you can pass the scope all the way up to the pelvi-ureteric junction and into the renal pelvis.

23. If you encounter stones, then they can either be fragmented using laser, electrohydraulic lithotripsy, or electrokinetic lithotripsy. If the stone is in the upper part of the ureter, then it may be flushed back into the kidney for subsequent extracorporeal lithotripsy. Try to avoid baskets in the upper part of the ureter, as this may cause ureteric injury. In order to fragment the stone you will need to remove the second guidewire, but keep the "safety" wire.

24. Other treatment or diagnostic procedures can be performed through the ureteroscope including obtaining urine for cytology, or treating ureteric strictures, although this is beyond the scope of this book.

25. If damage is suspected to the ureter or you are worried that post-operative edema will develop, then you can insert a stent over the safety wire after removal of the ureteroscope scope, using a cystoscope (*see* Chapter 29).

Complications

Occasional complications include:

- Mild burning or bleeding on passing urine for short period after operation
- Urinary retention, necessitating temporary insertion of a bladder catheter
- Insertion of ureteric stent, requiring a further procedure to remove it
- Failure to pass ureteroscope, if the ureter is narrow

Rare complications include:

- Damage to ureter with need for open operation or a nephrostomy tube inserted from the back to allow any leaks to heal

- Kidney damage or infection, requiring further treatment
- Later scarring or stricture of the ureter, requiring further procedures

The patient should also be warned that there is no guarantee of cure, as this procedure is often diagnostic only and if cancer is found then additional therapy may be required.

Reference

1. The British Association of Urological Surgeons (Consent forms). http://www.baus. org.uk. Date accessed: May 25, 2007.

Index

Printed in the United States of America